Help for Your Headache

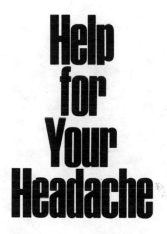

Help for Your Headache

by Edward Edelson

Introduction by Seymour Diamond, M.D.

Published in association with *Parade* magazine.

GROSSET & DUNLAP
A NATIONAL GENERAL COMPANY
Publishers   *New York*

Introduction

ALL PHYSICIANS, NO matter what their speciality, are called upon to treat patients with headache. Because headache is such a common symptom, the complaints of these patients are often ignored or minimized much to the chagrin and added worries of the sufferer. Headache is the only symptom to which a medical association is devoted: the American Association for the Study of Headache. In this organization a group of physicians has joined together to encourage research and to discuss treatment possibilities of various headache problems. Most discussions on headache begin with the statement that it is merely a symptom and not a disease. To the physician it should always be a symptom, the cause of which needs intensive exploration.

As a physician who for the past eight years has devoted most of his efforts to research and treatment of headache, I feel honored to write the introduction to this excellent discussion of headache. This book has been very adequately oriented for the layman's understanding of headache problems. The headache patient who was repeated severe pain will have hidden fears that he may have a brain tumor or an incurable illness. I have found, and this book illustrates, that the majority of the headache problems are not of such a nature. Careful and complete exploration by the physician in the form of a careful history, physical and neurological examination and the necessary laboratory and other tests, will usually enable a diagnosis to be made. The reassurance to the patient that a permanent or fatal disability is not present may be all that is necessary to help many of the sufferers. Most sufferers of head pain can be helped once a diagnosis is made.

The ideal disease from a physician's point of view should have a single cause, a short duration, and a rapid effective cure. This is not usually the case with headache problems. In our Headache Clinic at Mount Sinai Hospital and Medical Center, Bernard J. Baltes, my Co-Director, and myself, will exhaustively go over a patient's history and neurological examination to find the etiology, as do other doctors in serious pursuit of the reasons behind headache pain. Very often we have found that our patients are suffering from a depressive illness from which they have a constant headache and accompanying sleep disturbance with early and frequent awakening. Many headache problems are of a mixed nature, such as depression accompanying migraine. The detective ability of a Sherlock Holmes may be necessary in some instances to find the key to the headache problem. Medical research has usually been concentrated on the "killing diseases" (stroke, heart disease, cancer, etc.). Headache does not come under this category. It is encouraging that migraine and other causes of head pain are now the subject of a great deal of research. Such organizations as the British Migraine Association and the National Headache Foundation in the United States are now dedicating funds and efforts toward research of headache problems. This book should serve as a valuable reference to headache sufferers and their families and enable them to better understand their problems.

Seymour Diamond, M.D.,
Clinical Assistant Professor of Neurology,
The Chicago Medical School; Co-Director of the
Headache Clinic, Mount Sinai Hospital & Medical
Center; Secretary and Program Chairman, American
Association for the Study of Headache; and
Chairman, Department of Family Medicine, St. Joseph
Hospital, Chicago, Illinois.

Contents

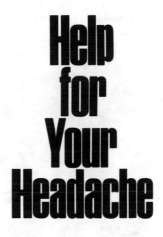

Help for Your Headache

1.

An Introduction
to Headache

THE TITLE OF this chapter is misleading, because no one
really needs an introduction to headache. Of all the ailments that have afflicted the human race through the mil-
lenia, headache probably is the one that has caused the
most pain to the most people. And headaches probably
have prompted as many quack cures and inflated promises
as the mind of man is capable of producing.

No one knows who had the first headache. But we do
have medical records indicating that head pains have
troubled mankind since the earliest days of civilization.
For example, the oldest complete medical book known to
exist is the Ebers Papyrus, which dates back 3,500 years.
This compendium of ancient medical advice, found in the
long-dead Egyptian city of Thebes, mentions "a sickness
of half the head"—a clear reference to migraine.

The ancient inhabitants of what is now Peru left even
more vivid evidence implicating headache as one of their
medical problems. Skulls found in ancient Peruvian

1

graveyards occasionally have neat round holes drilled in them—holes that were made while the person was alive. This technique, called trephination, can be performed with reasonable safety even under relatively primitive conditions. Some modern physicians conjecture that these Peruvian trephinations may sometimes have been performed in an attempt to ease the throbbing pain of headache that occasionally seems to the sufferer to threaten to split the skull wide open.

To some extent, ancient history is being repeated today. American physicians estimate that half the people who walk into their offices complain of headaches. Virtually every adult American has had a headache—when the children were crying, when deadline pressures mount unbearably, on the morning after a night of overdoing it. But for an estimated one in twelve adult Americans, headache is more than just an occasional nuisance. These people suffer from chronic recurring headaches—pain that comes again and again, often without warning, and lasts for hours or days.

Americans spend about $300 million a year on popular, often self-prescribed remedies for headaches. Often those remedies are little more effective than, but not as drastic as, the holes drilled in skulls in long-ago Peru. But there is a major difference between what ancient medicine and the modern physician can do for headaches. Physicians today have an arsenal of drugs and techniques that can bring relief to the great majority of headache sufferers.

That arsenal has been forged in the medical research laboratory. Over the past few decades, painstaking experiments have given physicians an increasingly clear picture of the causes of headaches. With that knowledge has come a variety of new headache-fighting methods. Not all the answers are known by any means. But the chances of finding headache relief today are better than ever before in history, thanks to the continuing research effort.

Perhaps the leading figure in headache research was the

late Dr. Harold G. Wolff of Cornell Medical College in New York. In years of careful experimentation, Dr. Wolff accumulated vast amounts of knowledge about headaches. Many of the techniques he used were invented by him, and still are used by headache researchers. Medical scientists have gone far beyond the knowledge gathered by Dr. Wolff and his coworkers, but it was the pioneering work that made advances possible.

Probably the most startling fact to come out of that research concerns the mechanism of headache pain. Working with patients undergoing brain operations, Dr. Wolff established the amazing fact that it isn't the brain that hurts during a headache. The brain cannot feel any pain, even though it has billions of nerve cells, because none of its nerve cells have the ability to transmit pain messages.

But obviously something *is* hurting up there during a headache. What is it?

That depends. Mostly it depends on the type of headache that the patient has. For even though most nonmedical people lump all headaches together, physicians know there are many different varieties; discovering the precise kind of headache that troubles a patient often requires acute medical detective work on the doctor's part.

But basically headaches can be classified under three categories, on the basis of the cause of the pain.

One group of headaches arises from the blood vessels of the head. Everyone knows that the body has an elaborate, complex system of arteries and veins to bring blood to every living cell. The blood carries oxygen and other nutriments to the cells and carries away waste products. The brain's blood supply is especially essential, because of the brain's unusual need for oxygen. The billions of nerve cells making up the tiny but efficient computer that every human being is born with can go without oxygen for just about four minutes. After that, brain cells begin to die, and nothing can bring them back to life again.

That means that the blood vessels supplying the brain must expand to carry more blood when the necessity arises. One kind of headache occurs when the blood vessels in the head expand too much for too long. There are plenty of pain-feeling nerves (called sensory nerves) in the walls of the blood vessels. As these walls expand, the sensory nerves are stretched, and they start transmitting pain messages. That pain can be felt for days at a time. When it is felt, someone is having a headache.

Because the blood vessels are called the "vascular system," headaches caused by problems with the blood vessels are called vascular headaches. The most common kind of vascular headache is migraine, which is perhaps the most complex headache. Physical troubles with the blood vessels of the head can also cause vascular headaches. These troubles—which, happily, tend to be rare—include brain tumors, meningitis, and the ballooning out of a weak section of a blood vessel wall, which goes under the medical name of an aneurysm.

A second type of headache comes from the muscles. All the body's physical work depends on muscle activity. Every time you pick up a package, walk down the street, or just turn your head, muscles are contracting and relaxing to do the work. Because muscles work, they need a constant supply of oxygen and nutriments, and constant removal of the waste products produced by their efforts. Ordinarily, the blood vessels supplying a given muscle perform both functions, bringing oxygen and carrying away waste products as the muscles contract and then relax.

It's when a muscle contracts and stays contracted for a long period of time that trouble begins. Continued contraction begins to cut down the body supply to that muscle, so that the muscle has less oxygen brought to it and begins to accumulate waste products. The result of prolonged contraction is pain—a steady, dull pain, compared to the throbbing pain typical of vascular headaches.

You can feel this kind of pain in your head if the muscles

of your head are kept contracted for too long. Unfortunately, the biological inheritance of the human race includes a built-in invitation to this kind of contraction. It's something of an instinct. When an animal is alert, it lifts its head, tensing head and neck muscles. People tend to do the same thing. On the ball field, for instance, when something goes wrong the cry is, "Heads up!"

When man had to keep an eye out for predatory animals, the heads-up position was useful. Today, when worries about wild animals have been replaced by worries about the household budget and the job, the old instinct no longer serves its intended purpose. But many people still react in the old way to tensions: they contract their head and neck muscles without realizing that they're doing it. In this case, heads-up posture just produces headache.

This kind of headache goes under a two-edged name: tension headache. Physicians use the word "tension" to refer to the contracted, or tense, state of the muscles. Most nonmedical people are likely to think that the term refers to the mental tension that causes the muscles to contract, producing the headache.

In most cases, either meaning is accurate. But other factors aside from simple nervous tension can cause tension headaches. Poor lighting, arthritis, and drafty rooms, among other things, can produce muscle contractions that lead to headache. Increasingly, physicians studying tension headaches find that depression is a major factor in causing them.

The third type of headache is caused by direct irritation of nerves in the head. These headaches include the sharp, jabbing pains of tic doloreux, the dull headache, accompanied by dizziness, of Meniere's Disease, and the steady pain caused by neuritis (inflammation of a nerve), by injury to a nerve, by a growth on a nerve or by other conditions that cause similar abnormalities.

Headaches caused by nerve abnormalities affect many

fewer people than do vascular and tension headaches. One leading expert, Dr. Arnold P. Friedman, head of the world-famous Headache Unit at Montefiore Hospital in New York, estimates that 90 per cent of all headaches seen by physicians are vascular or tension head-aches—occasionally in combination.

This threefold division of headaches just barely begins to give an idea of the complexity of the subject. There are many different types and subtypes of headache within each of these three classifications. Doctors don't always agree on how to classify headaches, but they keep trying. One of the most authoritative efforts was made several years ago by a committee of experts, with Dr. Friedman as chairman.

The committee was appointed by the National Institute of Neurological Diseases and Stroke, the federal agency whose responsibilities include headache research. It's important to note that the committee's work was more than just an exercise in neatness; that work has paid benefits for headache patients.

As the committee noted in its final report, careful distinctions between the different types of headache can help doctors diagnose specific cases, and pick the best treatment for those cases. Since a drug that performs miracles for one kind of headache may be useless or even harmful against other types, diagnosing the headache is one of the most important things a physician can do. This classification helps make diagnosis more precise. And it also illustrates the surprisingly large number of things that can go wrong inside the head, starting the headache cycle.

Here, in simplified form, is the committee's classification:

1. Vascular headaches of the migraine type. The committee listed five different headaches in this group; other experts list only three. These headaches are discussed in detail in Chapter Three.

2. Muscle-contraction headaches, which are also called tension headaches. These will be discussed in Chapter Two.

3. Combined headache: vascular and muscle contraction. Migraine and tension headaches can go together, as described in Chapter Three.

4. Headaches of nasal vasomotor reaction. That complicated name means that something causes congestion and edema (collection of excess fluid) in the sensitive tissues that line the nasal area, leading to headache. See Chapters five and six.

5. Headache of delusional, conversional or hypochondriacal states. These headaches are literally "all in your head"—headaches that people simply think themselves into having. It's easy, if you try hard enough. See Chapter Two.

At this point in its listing, the committee paused to note that the first five types of headache are those most commonly seen by the physician. This should be a relatively minor point for the patient, except for one thing: that fact serves to ease what can be a major worry. Many people who suffer from recurring headaches are prone to worry about the possibility that they have brain tumors. For those people, the word from the experts is—relax. Tumor is a relatively uncommon cause of headache. (But that does not mean that a headache sufferer can cheerfully avoid seeing a physician. Even though the chances of having a tumor are small, it's wise to consult a physician about any recurring headache.)

Having made that point, the committee resumed its listing:

6. Nonmigrainous vascular headaches. Two types are listed: vascular headaches caused by infections, and those caused by "miscellaneous causes." These disorders include such unrelated causes as carbon monoxide, chemicals that cause the blood vessels to stretch, reaction to a concussion, low levels of blood sugar, and high blood pressure—a miscellaneous list, indeed.

The one thing they have in common is their pain-causing effect on the blood vessels of the head.

7. Traction headaches. These are caused by disorders that produce traction—stretching and pushing—of structures in the head. Among these causes are tumors, hematomas (blood clots, usually caused by injury), abscesses, and swelling of the brain.

8. Headache produced by cranial inflammation. Infections and other disorders can cause structures in the head to become inflamed, and headache is the result.

9-13. Headaches due to diseases of the eyes, the ears, the nose, the sinuses, the teeth, and other structures of the head and neck. This obviously is a broad class (or group of classes). All these headaches have the same basic cause—something goes wrong in or near the head (an injury, an infection, or a growth, most likely), and the result is painful stimulation of the head nerves.

14. Cranial neuritides (a word that is simply the plural of neuritis). This can be caused by injury, tumor, or inflammation.

15. Cranial neuralgias. For the patient, the difference between neuritis and neuralgia is this: in neuritis, the pain is likely to be more or less continuous. In neuralgia, the pain often is swift, stabbing, and of short duration, although it comes back later.

That completes the list. If you examine it, you'll notice that there's still another way to classify these headaches, into two groups this time. One group of headaches is caused by what physicians call an organic problem—a physical difficulty, such as an infection or a tumor, that causes pain. The second group has no organic basis; instead, its origin is emotional. While the number of headaches of organic origin in the list is large, in actual practice physicians find that most headaches arise from emotional tension.

To cure a headache of organic origin, the doctor treats the underlying condition. Treating the other kind of headache is trickier. Drugs can do much to help the headache sufferer, but physicians usually find that some understanding of the emotional basis of the headache is vital to truly effective treatment.

Another classification groups the same headaches somewhat differently. This classification was made by the American Association for the Study of Headache, the only medical organization in the country that is devoted to the study of a symptom, not a disease. The physicians who favor this classification believe that the one already listed may be too complex, and therefore may cause unnecessary complications for the general practitioner who is trying to help a headache patient.

There are only three main headings in this classification scheme. The first is vascular headaches, which are listed as follows:

A. Migraine
    1. Classic
    2. Hemiplegic
    3. Ophthalmologic
B. Cluster (histamine)
C. Toxic
D. Hypertensive.

The different varieties of migraine headaches usually are of more interest to the physician than to the patient, whose only concern is getting the pain stopped, no matter what its name may be. Cluster headaches are discussed in Chapter Four, toxic headaches in Chapter Twelve and hypertensive headaches in Chapter Nine.

The second heading is muscle contraction headaches:

A. Anxiety and Tension
B. Depressive equivalents and conversion reactions
C. Cervical arthritis

D. Chronic myositis (muscle inflammation)

And the third heading is traction and inflammatory headaches:

A. Mass lesions (tumors, etc.)
B. Diseases of the eye, ear, nose, throat and teeth
C. Cranial neuralgia
D. Allergy
E. Infection
F. Arteritis and Phlebitis

As can be seen, both classifications list the same headaches, with the same causes. The object in classifying headaches is to enable physicians to identify the precise headache in any particular case, so that the right treatment can be given. This last classification is primarily the work of Dr. Donald J. Dalessio, head of the Division of Neurology at the Scripps Clinic and Research Foundation, La Jolla, California.

In practice, none of these classifications is as precise as it seems. Diagnosing a headache is not a matter of running the finger down a list and picking the right category. Headaches with vastly different causes can resemble each other closely. And headache patients often suffer from more than one type of headache. That is why physicians are fond of quoting a statement made by one expert: "If I wanted to show a medical student how difficult it is to practice medicine, I would give him a headache patient to manage."(It should be mentioned that the statement was made before modern researchers made their great advances.)

From the patient's point of view, a headache offers a different kind of challenge—the challenge of maintaining civility and sanity in the face of crippling pain that goes on for hour after agonizing hour. The person with chronic recurring headaches needs all the help he can get, and part of that help comes from knowing the facts about headaches, which can be quite reassuring.

So to start with, here are three basic facts about headaches. There are some exceptions to all three, but they still are true in the great majority of cases.

Fact One: A headache is a symptom, not a disease.

Surprisingly, this means that a headache can actually be good for you, because it gives you notice that something is wrong. After all, pain makes us react in ways that are beneficial; it can drive us to our dentist, for instance, when we have a toothache.

Any headache sufferer should keep this in mind: In some cases, headache is a signal of disease. For other people, chronic headaches are an indication of something that isn't quite right in the way they live. Anyone who suffers from recurring headaches should check with the family doctor, to try to determine what is wrong. It could be nothing more than a poorly prescribed pair of eyeglasses, or it could be an emotional crisis. Whatever it is, the person suffering from such headaches owes it to himself to find out what's wrong.

In nine cases out of ten, there is no underlying organic cause for chronic headaches. In that tenth case, there is something physically wrong with the patient; in a few cases, whatever is wrong may require immediate attention to prevent serious consequences. A person who has frequent, recurring headaches is making a major mistake if he or she does not seek medical treatment.

Fact Two: Most headache patients think themselves into trouble.

Of course, that's a gross oversimplification; some headaches are unavoidable, no matter how well-adjusted a person is. But the fact remains that the greatest single cause of headache is emotional tension.

There's a good way and a bad way to tell this to the person with headaches. The bad way is to say, "You're really responsible for all your own problems." This is an excellent method of increasing tension, thus increasing the possibility of future headaches. The other way, which is both more helpful and more accurate, is to tell the headache patient that he can do a lot to help himself. A good

11

many tense people are unaware of their tensions; often, they are so accustomed to tension that they regard it as a normal way of life. Understanding that tension exists is the first step toward relieving that tension.

The most important exception to this rule is migraine. Physicians know that there is a strong emotional element in many cases of migraine. But recent research has shown that migraine is a condition that can be passed down from generation to generation in a family. The emotions do play a role, but the organic element is present as well.

Fact Three: No one ever died from a headache.

This may sound like a frivolous statement, but it is important. Persons in the throes of a chronic headache may feel as if they are dying, and they often worry about the possibility that a serious disease is upon them. However, aside from some kinds of migraine that can cause permanent damage to some nerves, headaches usually do no harm beyond the pain and suffering of the moment.

Again, there's a bad way and a good way to get this across. The bad way is to tell a headache sufferer that there's no need to worry and no need to see a physician. The good way is to have a physician assure the patient, after careful examination, that there is no serious organic complaint behind the headache.

To repeat: a headache is a symptom that something is wrong. Anyone suffering from chronic headaches should see a doctor. But the headache sufferer can take comfort from knowing that the odds are on his side as far as the possibility of a potentially fatal disease is concerned.

There's one final fact that should be stated: the headache patients shouldn't expect miracle cures. So much has been written about the miracles performed by modern drugs that many patients despair when they don't get instant relief. Some of these patients thereupon begin trying one nostrum after another, switching from compound to compound in search of the impossible. It's a practice that is encouraged by the insistent advertising campaigns mounted by some manufacturers of over-the-counter headache products. Many of these products are fine, if used in moderation for the right reasons (although few of them offer any significant advantages over plain old reliable aspirin). But people who are looking for happiness in a bottle of pills seldom find it.

Relief is possible for the great majority of patients suffering from chronic recurrent headaches; experts estimated that three of every four patients can get more or less permanent headache relief under the care of a competent physician. Drugs do play an important role in many cases. But the personal attention and counseling of the physician is an equally important element. The type and number of drugs to be taken, the dosage and the timing usually can be set only after careful analysis by the physician. A patient who tries to be his own doctor in a case like this is just asking for trouble.

When a physician takes on a headache patient, he prepares himself for several office sessions of probing questions; it takes valuable time, but the physician knows that there is no substitute for complete knowledge of the headache and the person who has it. So it's only fair for the patient to make the same kind of commitment. He can help the physician—and himself—by understanding the nature of headaches and his own nature better. This book is written to help make that process of understanding easier.

2.

Tension Headache

JOHN WAS A good headwaiter and proud of it. Night after night, ushering celebrities to their tables in a fashionable New York restaurant, he was always smiling, always affable, even under the most hectic circumstances. But day after day, he lived in dread of the headaches that seemed to clamp down on his head. They were becoming more frequent and more severe, like a steel band drawn ever tighter around his forehead.

Ann was a secretary who had worked for years for the same executive and was suddenly transferred to the secretarial pool. Instead of easy-going treatment from a boss who liked and appreciated her work, she got a multitude of hurry-up assignments from executives who hardly knew her name and who were quick to criticize any error. Mondays were the worst, because the secretarial pool was short-staffed that day. But Sundays were the days she dreaded. They were likely to be days of headache—a dull boring pain that seemed to press steadily on

14

her head and neck.

Ethel was a middle-aged housewife whose husband barely earned a decent living. Her children were grown up and out of the house. For years, she had been in bad health, never quite sick but never quite completely healthy. An operation had helped her stomach trouble, but now she was bothered by headaches that often were accompanied by dizziness and nausea. She had tried almost every compound in the drugstore without success; now she was thinking about taking her problems to her family doctor.

When these three patients came to their physicians, the diagnosis in each case was fairly easy to make: tension headache caused by emotional problems. In other cases the diagnosis is not so simple—the emotional problem that causes the headache may not be so close to the surface, there may be organic factors involved to confuse the issue, or the type of pain described by the patient may point to a different kind of headache.

Nevertheless, physicians find that tension headaches probably are the most common kind seen in medical practice. That's because few people are free of the kind of emotional conflicts that cause such headaches. The head-waiter's straining to appear cheerful while his hostility was kept bottled up, the secretary's dread of another week of dull, repetitive work, were easy for the informed eye and ear of the surgeon to detect. But sometimes the trouble is deep beneath the surface: a middle-aged man worrying about his virility, a young matron whose teen-age daughter is running around in fast company, a college freshman worrying about tests and term papers—all these headache sufferers may not even realize that they are in emotional turmoil.

They also may not realize that they are tightening up on the muscles of the neck and head. Even strong contractions of these muscles may remain below the level of conscious awareness. And the pain caused by these contractions can spread far from its source. So when a headache begins, the patient has no explanation for it.

But the physician knows what to look for. There is a typical tension headache that leaves its tell-tale signs.

Unlike migraine headaches, which often signal their arrival beforehand, a tension headache comes on with little or no warning. The patient usually finds it hard to tell the doctor exactly where the pain is, but often there is a feeling of having a tight band compressed around the forehead. (That feeling is caused by contraction of scalp muscles.) The headache won't awaken the patient in the middle of the night, but it may be the first thing that the patient is aware of upon awakening. Sometimes—as in the secretary's case—it comes on a fairly regular schedule, occasionally even daily. It can last for a few hours, or for days on end. Nausea, weakness, irritability, and dizziness may accompany the headache. In some severe cases, the headache sufferer may feel as if his neck muscles are knotted up, which is close to the actuality. The pain is dull and steady, not throbbing, and it tends to be most intense at the back of the neck and the center of the forehead. Aspirin or another over-the-counter headache product may help for a while, but the headaches recur in spite of all the drugs the patient takes.

Many physicians draw a distinction between simple tension headaches and psychogenic headaches; they speak of "conversion" headaches and "hypochondriacal" headaches. These distinctions are valuable to physicians chiefly because they help define how deep-rooted the problem is. For the secretary, for example, tension headaches were a response to a situation that was fairly easy to correct. But the housewife's problem was much more deeply rooted in a whole life style. Although the basic physical and emotional mechanisms of the two women's headaches are similar, the two cases require essentially different approaches on the part of the physician.

But there is a common thread that can be discerned in many headache patients who are driven to see their physicians by unending pain. That thread is depression.

Says Dr. Seymour Diamond, codirector of the Headache Clinic at Chicago's Mount Sinai Hospital and Medical Center:

"It's been my observation that people with simple tension headache don't come to see the doctor. What is often described as tension is really depression. Tension headaches can usually be relieved by aspirin, but depression headaches require more careful handling and different drugs, notably the antidepressants."

Dr. Diamond has observed that such headaches usually occur in two time periods during any given day: from 4 p.m. to 8 p.m. and from 4 a.m. to 8 a.m. "These are usually the periods of the greatest and sometimes the most silent family crises," he points out. "It may be the time early in the morning when the depressed patient awakens and his fantasies of warfare with the members of his family or his work conflicts are manifested. In discussion with the depressed patient we find that his headaches occur when he leaves the quiet atmosphere of the office for a weekend at home. It often coincides with restful interpersonal situations in which the sufferer feels compelled to appear comfortable, relaxed and agreeable, although he is struggling to repress his resentment toward someone whom he is expected to love and respect."

There are other symptoms that usually go along with these headaches, Dr. Diamond finds—sleep disturbances, including insomnia and early awakening; loss of appetite, often accompanied by severe weight loss; and a decrease of sexual activity that may arouse fear of impotence in men and frigidity in women. Obviously, what started as a psychological problem can become a major physical disturbance requiring careful treatment.

In any headache, the physician has two aims: first to provide relief for existing pain as quickly as possible, and then to prevent the headache from recurring. Both aims go hand in hand, but the patient is naturally interested in getting rid of his pain.

There are a large number of drugs that physicians use to attack pain directly. Aspirin is the most widely used. It is both safe and effective, and careful studies under controlled conditions indicate that the relief it gives is as good as that given by more expensive pain-killing compounds, at least for most people. In many cases, the physician may prescribe a pain-killer other than aspirin, because he believes it may be better for an individual patient. Or he may prescribe a drug that combines aspirin or another pain-killer with ingredients that relax muscles or help calm the stomach.

Other drugs can provide relief in different ways. As has been mentioned, in about half the patients suffering from tension headaches, depression is a real factor; not only does it make the pain seem worse than it is, but it also prevents the patient from coming to grips with his problems. In these cases, the physician may prescribe an antidepressant drug to break the cycle of anxiety and sleeplessness that helps perpetuate the headaches.

Needless to say, the headache patient shouldn't take it on himself to decide which drugs are best for him. In our pill-conscious society, almost anyone will be ready to offer a tranquillizer, an antidepressant or a similar drug to a friend who seems to be in need of one. But because of the emotional element in these headaches, such self-medication can be risky. When a physician prescribes a tranquillizer or other drug, he often will limit their use to a specific period of time, keeping the patient under careful observation. "The need for careful observation is obvious," notes Dr. Arnold P. Friedman, "for the drugs are capable of producing marked side effects, both physical and mental." In short, with proper medical supervision, drugs can provide the help the patient wants so desperately.

Aside from drugs, there are other tools in the physicians' employ. One major objective is to increase the flow of blood to the area of tense muscles, thus striking directly at the physical cause of the headache. Heat and massage can do a lot; something as simple as a hot shower directed at the back of the neck or a long, soothing soak in a hot tub can start to relax muscles and ease the pain. Wet heat is regarded as more helpful than dry heat, because it penetrates deeper. But a heating pad or hot-water bottle at the back of the neck or on the forehead can help provide relief. Gentle massage of the tense muscles, particularly those at the back of the neck, or the use of vibrating devices to loosen the muscles can also help.

A treatment that some physicians may try is the injection of drugs into what they call "trigger points" of the body. These trigger points are spots where the knotted muscles are worst; they are even painful to the touch. Trigger points are found in the grooves of the neck muscles and in the brow. An injection of an anesthetic in these points often can relieve pain; some physicians may prefer to inject a steroid drug. This is a specialized procedure, however, and not every physician is willing to do it.

While he works to ease the immediate pain, the physician will undertake an even more important assignment: determining the cause of the recurring headaches so they can be prevented. This means first of all taking a detailed medical history, asking a host of questions about the patient's general health, now and in the past. The physician will want to know what past illnesses have been, if there is a history of headache in the family, and a lot of information about the headaches—when they began, how often they occur, where the pain is felt, whether any past treatment has been successful, and so on. He'll probably also perform a physical examination to add to the information gathered in his questioning. The more serious the headaches, the more intensive the history-taking and examination is likely to be.

Along the way, the physician probably will start asking a lot of what many patients regard as highly personal questions. Patients shouldn't take umbrage at these questions. They are asked to fulfill a dictum expressed by Dr.

Friedman: "The secret of successful treatment of the patient with tension headache can be summed up in one phrase: treat the whole patient."

The medical history and the physical examination tell the physician whether or not there is an organic cause, such as arthritis, for the headaches. But physicians know that there isn't any organic reason for most headaches. Usually, the emotions are responsible for the aching head. And so the physician sets out patiently to find out what is troubling his patient.

The fancy name for this effort is psychotherapy—literally, treatment for the mind. But that term frightens many people, who identify it only with serious mental illness. As the family physician uses the term, psychotherapy can best be defined as an effort to make the patient understand the mental and emotional sources of his physical problem.

Physicians have always known that any person's emotional outlook can affect his health. In the past few decades, research has built up a detailed picture of the way that unhappiness, frustration, worry and anxiety can alter the body's physical activity. The link leads from the brain to the hormones to the nervous system to the muscles. In a simplified way, the scientific picture is this: most hormones are produced (or not produced) under the control of the body's "master gland," the pituitary. This small gland, which is located in the middle of the skull, produces its hormones in response to signals from the brain. Other effects of mental processes are more direct, disturbing the process of digestion and, as we have seen, contracting some muscles abnormally. In short, anyone who worries enough will soon have some real medical problems to worry about.

When the physician starts asking his gently probing questions, he is out to get all the information he can about the emotional life of his patient. Since he is starting from scratch, he will follow up almost any lead. For example, he will want to know when headaches occur. If it is on a regular schedule—as with the secretary whose Sundays were ruined by tension headaches—the physician will follow up with questions aimed at ferreting out the periodic event that causes the headaches. If headaches strike with no apparent regularity, the physician may become interested in the last bad headache his patient had. His questions may sound odd: What did you do the night before? What were you intending to do the next day? Were you expecting any visit from relatives? Did anything unusual happen at home? On the job? They don't sound like medical questions at all. But obviously, any question that helps get to the root of the problem is a help.

The physician will also start to ask about the patient's life in general. Most of us are worried about the same things—money, the children, health, the job. In what may seem more like a conversation than a medical interview, the physician will ask about all these things. Again, he'll be trying to get to the root of the problem—the worry or worries that cause the headaches to keep coming back.

Often, this will be going on while the patient is still being treated for relief of pain. Many physicians prefer to have a series of relatively brief appointments, perhaps no more than ten minutes at a time, during which they can check up on the progress of drug therapy and gather the clues that eventually will reveal the cause of the problem.

It's obvious that for many patients, this is no quick process. Physicians are prepared to see a patient many times, finding out a little more each time, until they finally know the whole story. This can be one of the delicate processes in medical practice, for the patient as well as the physician. Some problems are so oppressive that people won't even admit they exist. Even though the doctor may know what the problem is after a brief time, his job is to make the patient realize it without jolting the patient into extra trouble.

21

"Over the long term," says Dr. Henry H. Garner of the Chicago Medical School, "the emphasis has got to be on, not the medication, not, 'How is your headache today?', but 'What is happening to your life today?' and 'Can you do without this medication?' "

In this psychotherapy, the doctor's aim is to help the patient help himself. In the case of the headwaiter, for example, the physician saw his patient periodically for months. During that time, the waiter talked about many things—not only his job, but his unhappy childhood, his hostilities and tensions at home. All his life, he said, he had kept his emotions bottled up, priding himself on his ability to carry on with a smile even though he was boiling inside. Under the physician's understanding care, the waiter came to realize that it was necessary for him to express his emotions more. As he found acceptable outlets for his anger, the headwaiter also found that he was getting fewer headaches, and that his headaches were milder.

Interestingly, nothing had changed outwardly. The waiter still had rude customers or surly waiters to handle at work and a standard quota of normal worries at home. But his mental life had changed: he knew now what caused his headaches. And that understanding was enough to give him significant relief from what had been crippling pain.

No physician will be able to end his patient's nonmedical problems. But a doctor can help a patient understand that those problems are not unusual, and that it is the patient's attitude toward everyday, essentially manageable troubles that leads to headaches.

Sometimes, of course, the situation changes. The secretary's Sunday headaches faded away after she went back to work as another executive's girl Friday. But the housewife with the low-earning husband and the troubled attitude toward life could find no such easy escape from her problems, real and imagined. Fortunately, she had an understanding family physician. After a few visits in which she talked constantly about her headaches, her bad stomach and her monetary problems, the physician began to chat about her children. Both a son and a daughter were doing well, even though they showed no appreciation for their parents' sacrifices. Letters to the children by the physician increased the number of visits they paid to their mother. Those visits greatly improved the patient's morale. Eventually the physician could make the housewife see that she wasn't much worse off financially than many other people. The headaches never really disappeared, but they have diminished.

When worries are real, the physician may turn to non-medical sources of help—the church, or social service agencies, which can help deal with specific problems. In some cases, the physician can help simply by assuring that patient that there is no organic disease, such as a brain tumor to worry about. But in most cases of tension headaches, the battle must be won or lost by the patient, even though the physician may provide significant help. By understanding his own mental processes, a headache patient can determine the amount of pain he will suffer in the future.

3.

Migraine Headache

FEW CONDITIONS HAVE a longer medical history than migraine headaches. As has been mentioned, the oldest medical book known probably mentions it. It was Galen, one of the greatest physicians of antiquity (he lived in the second century after Christ), who gave the condition a name. He called it "hemicrania," which means "one-sided headache." Over the centuries, the term evolved gradually to hemigrania, emigrania, migrainia, megrim, and finally migraine.

While patients are likely to call any severe recurring headache migraine, the physician uses the term to refer to a fairly precisely defined condition. This is more than just a semantic issue, because other types of headache that can be mistaken for migraine can't be helped by the kind of treatment that gives relief to many migraine sufferers. Often, however, the migraine attack is unmistakable.

The first stage of the migraine attack starts before the

head pain begins. A migraine attack almost invariably gives notice that it is on the way, although the warning signs may be difficult for the patient to detect. In about 10 per cent or more of all cases, there will be visual disturbances: double vision, difficulty in getting the eyes focussed, temporary partial blindness or even a dazzling display of colored lights, spots or lines. These usually occur about half an hour before the pain starts. In other cases, the warning signs will be more vague and will stretch back for a longer period before the onset of pain. Many patients experience nausea and vomiting before the headache begins. Others will notice they have speech difficulties, strange skin sensations, or sensitivity to noise or light. Still others will feel vaguely uneasy or irritable and unable to work. Some people find that their efficiency increases strangely on the day before an attack; a housewife may briskly clean the whole house or a businessman may go speedily through a pile of correspondence. Some people may begin urinating more frequently.

Sometimes the migraine patient will have vividly real hallucinations preceding the attack. The occurrence of these visions provides a fascinating medical sidelight on a book that is a classic for both adults and children. Lewis Carroll, who wrote *Alice in Wonderland*, was a migraine sufferer who is believed to have experienced hallucinations as part of his attacks. Some headache experts believe that those hallucinations were woven into his writings. So when an adult sits down to read this charming book to a child, part of the enjoyment may stem, ironically enough, from the pain suffered by the author nearly a century ago.

The next stage is the onset of pain, the intense, throbbing pain that migraine patients dread. It may take several hours for the pain to build to a peak; after that, it will continue at the same level for as long as twelve to eighteen hours. As the ancient name implies, the pain of migraine usually effects just one side of the head, but not always

25

the same side, and occasionally the entire head. It is a throbbing pain, beating in time with the heart. Often, the nausea and vomiting that preceded the headache continue after the pain begins; sensitivity to light and noise may also continue. Diarrhea or excessive urination may add to the discomfort. But it is the beat, beat, beat of the pain that makes migraine so terrible to its victims.

But after a while, the nature of the pain changes. Instead of throbbing, it settles into a steady, dull ache. That may keep up for days, gradually giving away to pain in the neck and scalp that is reminiscent of a muscle contraction headache. When the pain finally fades away, it may be replaced by a brief feeling of well-being, which is followed by a slow recovery.

It is one of the great achievements of headache research that physicians can now explain, step by step, almost all the physical changes that produce every stage of the migraine headache. While the picture is not complete yet, the advances in research laboratories all over the world are going on—and each advance brings the promise of relief to more patients.

For example, it is generally agreed that many of the warning signs of the headache are caused by changes in the blood vessels inside the head. These vessels constrict, become narrower, slowing down the flow of blood. This apparently deprives key areas of the brain of the blood they need to function properly, and the result is the visual disturbances, speech difficulties, and all the other signs of an approaching attack.

But the actual pain is caused by a different kind of change in different blood vessels. It is known that migraine's throbbing pain begins when the arteries on the exterior of the head dilate—expand and stretch. This stretching stimulates the pain-feeling nerves in the artery walls; the headache is under way.

But after some hours, the persistent dilation of the arteries begins to affect them. Normally soft and flexible, the artery walls start to become more rigid and thicker. Excess fluid accumulates, and the nerves in the artery walls come under continuous pressure. In the process, the throbbing pain of the headache's first stage changes into a steady pain caused by the continuous stimulation of the nerves. The long-lasting pain may cause the sufferer's head and neck muscles to tighten up, so that the last painful hours of a migraine headache are really a muscle contraction headache. Finally comes the feeling of relief as the pain fades, and the recovery to normal.

This outline of a migraine headache was made by Dr. Wolff after years of research. Since his pioneering work, other researchers have begun to add enormous detail to the picture. Their work has led them into all the complexity of the human brain, the human body, and the human personality.

Among other things, they have found that most migraine headache patients are women. The reason for this is not completely understood, but the sexual differences are believed to have their root in the hormonal differences between men and women. Other phenomena of migraine, once equally puzzling, are better understood today.

For example, you may have noticed what seemed to be a contradictory explanation: in the warning stages of the headache, blood vessels constrict (become tighter). But when the pain begins, it is because other blood vessels have dilated (become looser). How can two such diametrically opposite reactions be involved in the same condition?

The attempt to answer that question led researchers to a group of chemicals that can affect the blood vessels, the muscles and the nerves of the body. These compounds now are in the forefront of modern medical research—not only because of their role in headache, but because they seem to play a fundamental role in the functioning and malfunctioning of the brain. Even if help for millions of headache sufferers were not involved, this research would still be fascinating.

Consider one of these chemicals, discovered in 1948, which has been named serotonin. Different researchers have found that the action of serotonin can vary in different parts of the body and even at different times in the same individual. To give just one example, serotonin can make some blood vessels dilate and other blood vessels constrict. That kind of activity, of course, fits right in with the "contradictory" effects that occur during a migraine headache.

Researchers have found in laboratory tests that both kinds of serotonin activity can be inhibited by a chemical named methysergide, of which much more will be heard later in this chapter. Methysergide turns out to be a close chemical relative of lysergic acid diethylamide, the LSD that so many young people now use to produce hallucinations. So there is a surprisingly short chain linking serotonin to the functioning of the brain; some researchers, in fact, believe that mental disorders may be caused by serotonin abnormalities in the brain.

What is all of this laboratory work doing to help headache patients? Well, it's logical to assume that if methysergide inhibits serotonin activity, and if serotonin is involved in migraine, then methysergide might help migraine patients. And indeed, methysergide does. The discovery that this drug could help migraine patients was first hailed as one of the most significant advances ever made in headache treatment. Marketed under the trade name Sansert by Sandoz Pharmaceuticals, methysergide has been taken daily by thousands of migraine sufferers to prevent attacks. More recently, however, there has been a trend away from methysergide because of the extremely severe side effects that can occur with its daily use. Methysergide remains a potent drug that can provide some patients with help when all else fails, but physicians who use it recommend that each patient should have a kidney X-ray at least twice a year and should

28

be checked by the physician on a week-to-week basis.

Methysergide's success would seem to clinch the case against serotonin as the villain in migraine. However, research indicates that the case isn't that simple. Other chemicals have been implicated in various stages of the migraine attack, and personality and emotional factors also play a large role in migraine. It is a complex puzzle that researchers are attempting to solve, but the promise of help for more headache patients spurs them on.

Serotonin, for example, isn't the only chemical that can affect the nerves and muscles; several others, related to it chemically, have similar effects. Further complicating the picture is the existence of a number of pain-causing compounds called the kinins, which are produced and released inside the body in response to some types of attack. Probably the best-known of these chemicals is histamine, the compound that is blamed for many of the annoying symptoms of the common cold and of allergies. Other kinins cause inflammation, which, it should be noted, involves dilation of blood vessels, among other things.

Why should the body make such troublesome stuff? Because inflammation is one method of fighting injuries; it sets loose repair mechanisms that eventually put things right. It's only when the mechanism goes haywire, as in allergy (an abnormal response to a harmless substance) that the kinins cause trouble. The belief now is that at least part of the migraine problem is due to a haywire reaction of that type.

That belief is based partially on the discovery at the site of migraine headaches of a close chemical relative of histamine. Christened neurokinin, this chemical has intriguing properties. Not only does it make the blood vessels more permeable, it also lowers the pain threshhold, so that a little bit of painful stimulation causes more pain. Neurokinin apparently is not responsible for the initial dilation of the artery walls that causes pain. But once that dilation begins, some unknown factor causes either the release of neurokinin from cells or its production by nearby cells. Once it is present, neurokinin seems to prolong the headache and make the pain worse. It is a completely local phenomenon, since neurokinin is found only in the immediate area of the headache pain. Blood samples taken from other parts of the patient's body contain no neurokinin at all.

It is obvious that the last word on the role of natural chemicals in migraine has not been said. In fact, this is one of the hottest areas of headache research. The success of methysergide has set scientists off on a methodical search for other chemicals in migraine and for chemicals to fight the pain-causing substances in the body. Several promising compounds have been found and are being tested; one or two even have been licensed for use overseas, where regulatory agencies are less strict about proof of safety than U. S. government officials. There is hope for more relief for more migraine sufferers through drug research.

But there is more to migraine than chemicals. Two other highly important factors that engage the interests of researchers are heredity and personality. The relationship of both heredity and personality is not absolutely clear, but few physicians doubt that there is such a relationship.

One of the first questions that any physician will ask a headache patient is whether there is a family history of migraine and other headaches. It is well established that a large proportion of migraine sufferers come from families where migraine is common. One researcher studied a number of families in which both husband and wife had migraine. He found that 83 per cent of the children of these parents had migraine attacks and 91 per cent of the parents had a family history of migraine. Similar studies have produced the same kind of results.

In the past, some physicians have denied that migraine is a physical condition that can be inherited; they explain the studies of inheritance by blaming the headaches on a "migraine personality." A parent with the "migraine personality," these physicians argue, is likely to bring up children in such a way that they, too, will develop the same sort of headaches, as will the children's children after them. Instead of a physical inheritance, these experts argued for an emotional inheritance as the reason for migraine families.

But in recent years, as knowledge of genetics (the science of inheritance) and of migraine has increased, this argument has tended to lose sway. Most headache experts now believe that children can inherit a physical tendency to migraine headaches. Dr. James W. Lance, of the University of New South Wales, Australia, put it in scientific terms at a 1970 symposium on headaches: "The present concept of migraine is that of a hereditary vascular instability which renders the individual susceptible to alteration in the level of humoral vasoactive substances (chemicals that affect the blood vessels), particularly serotonin."

In other words, Dr. Lance said, some people are unusually sensitive to changes in concentrations of chemicals such as serotonin. When the amount of serotinin decreases, these people suffer from unusual dilation of scalp arteries, which causes a migraine headache.

Genetic experts have tried to put this in even stricter biological terms. They know that every trait of every individual is governed by genes, small packets of information carried in the nucleus of all cells. It is entirely possible, these experts say, that such a thing as a "gene for migraine" exists, and that it is passed down, generation after generation, through certain families.

Does that mean that there's no hope for migraine sufferers, that they are doomed to have headaches all their lives, and that their children will suffer the same fate? The answer is a fairly definite no. For one thing, information about the genetic basis of migraine is far from complete; for example, the exact mode of inheritance and the specific abnormality that is inherited are not yet known. For another thing, the best information available indicates that what most migraine patients inherit is a *tendency* to develop the headaches, not a certainty of developing them. Whether or not a person has a headache seems to depend on any number of factors. And here is where personality comes in.

Not long ago, the existence of the migraine personality was accepted by a large number of physicians. Today they're not so sure, and many experts deny flatly that a migraine personality exists. There's no question that many migraine sufferers fit in the definition of the migraine personality: unusually sensitive, high-strung, compulsively perfectionist and unusually precise, often with strong feelings of hostility toward one's self for failing to meet self-set high standards of achievement. Some observers have detected a tendency toward migraine among intelligent, creative people whose striving for success leads to a rigid, anxious outlook toward friends and family.

Physicians even use this tendency as a tool for diagnosing migraine. One tell-tale sign is a long, detailed list of migraine attacks and all the various treatments that the patient has tried. When a patient walks in with such a list, the odds are that migraine is the problem. "Every headache patient we see with true migraine will come in to the office with a list," says one headache specialist.

Every physician has seen patients exactly like this who suffer the agonies of migraine. But every physician has also seen many patients with this type of personality who have never had a single migraine headache. Personality may be an important factor in many cases of migraine, but since it's possible to have the "migraine personality" without having migraine, the patient's outlook on life and the way he handles his problems obviously aren't the whole story.

It might be better if they were, because migraine would be relatively simple to treat if physicians just had to worry about a single factor, such as headache. Instead, research has shown that many, many different factors, chemical, emotional and other, play a part in the migraine syndrome. To give some examples:

Physicians studying individual patients sometimes find that they can trace migraine attacks to specific foods. The foods that are most commonly implicated are chocolate, dairy products, alcohol and citrus fruits. Several years ago, two British researchers, Edda Hanington and A. Murray Harper, set out to find the link between migraine and these foods. They found that a chemical called tyramine was present in large amounts in the foods that cause migraine.

That made sense, because tyramine turns out to be a member of the family of chemicals that affects nerves, muscles and blood vessels. Tests by the British experimenters showed that tyramine can cause blood vessels first to constrict and then to dilate—exactly the sequence of events that occurs in a migraine headache. Tyramine doesn't seem to work directly on the blood vessels; instead, it releases chemicals that do. So the connection between food and migraine is surprisingly direct.

In another British research project, Drs. J.N. Blau and D. A. Pyke in London studied thirty-six patients who had both migraine and diabetes. In five of those patients, they found that the migraine attacks had stopped with the onset of diabetes; several other patients noted that migraine attacks occurred only when they missed a meal.

The experimenters concluded that the key fact in these cases was the concentration of sugar in the blood. Diabetes increases the levels of blood sugar greatly—and for some people, at least, more sugar in the blood prevents migraine attacks. The researchers said that the sugar probably did not act directly, but had its effect on migraine because of its influence on the section of the nervous system that governs the blood vessels of the head. But the researchers were quick to add that blood sugar levels did not affect migraine attacks in every patient; other influences—including other diseases—were also at work.

One other tantalizing clue: some 80 per cent of women migraine sufferers stop having headaches during pregnancy, when the hormonal balance of the body changes drastically. That female sex hormones can affect migraine has been proven by studying women taking birth control pills, which contain artificial hormones. In addition, migraine headaches are connected to the menstrual cycle. In some women, the Pill can precipitate a migraine attack, or worsen one that is under way. To complete the picture, up to 75 per cent of female migraine patients get significant relief after the menopause, when their bodies' production of female sex hormones decreases sharply.

Once again, however, the picture is far from simple. The emotions seem to play a role as well as the hormones. "Financially insecure widows, unhappily married women and those with children who agitate them are not as apt to obtain this 'natural relief,'" notes Dr. Leonard L. Lovshin of the Cleveland Clinic. Attempts to treat migraine patients with hormone preparations have been far from an outstanding success.

Those are just a sample of the complications that turn up in a study of migraine. Do these complications mean that the treatment of migraine is beyond the powers of the average physician? Far from it. Indeed, each new complication reported by a researcher is actually a help. By adding to physicians' knowledge of this complex condition, the new information helps focus the attack on it. Today, most migraine patients can expect appreciable relief from their physicians' help.

As is the case with muscle contraction headache, the first concern of both patient and physician is to stop the pain; preventing new migraine attacks comes later. In fighting migraine, drugs are the first line of defense.

The most important drug used in treating migraine attacks is ergotamine tartrate, which was developed in 1932. But the medical history of this drug goes back much further. It first made its appearance as a menace, not a help. In times of famine, when people are forced to eat moldy grain, there have been outbreaks of poisoning, often severe enough to cause death; the symptoms include cramping pains of the arms and legs and gangrene, which can lead to loss of fingers and toes. The poisoning is caused by ergot, a fungus that grows on the moldy grain. It is this ergot, suitably tamed, that now helps headache sufferers.

Even before 1900, some physicians noted that ergot relieved migraine headaches. But they also noted that too often, migraine patients were stricken by the symptoms of ergot poisoning. Scientists began working on the problem of producing a form of ergot that would minimize these side effects. The result was ergotamine tartrate, which was made available in 1932 and has been a staple drug in the treatment of migraine ever since then.

Ergotamine, scientists have found, relieves migraine because it has a constricting effect on blood vessels, especially on the blood vessels of the scalp. (Recent research indicates that ergotamine also seems to counteract the effects of serotonin.) Since dilation of scalp arteries is the principle manifestation of migraine, ergotamine is an obvious weapon against migraine pains.

But to be effective, ergotamine must be taken at the right time during the headache attack: before the pain has built to its peak, and preferably during the warning stages. The best chance of preventing the attack is to get as much ergotamine as possible into the bloodstream, where it does its work. Injections are the best method of achieving that goal, but most patients cannot get to the doctor's office whenever a migraine attack is on the way, and so there are a number of other forms of ergotamine available: suppositories, liquids, mouth sprays and tablets. The physician will prescribe the form he thinks best.

Suppositories will be prescribed when possible, because they insure quick absorption of the drug. The intestine is honeycombed with blood vessels that will absorb ergotamine with little delay. But there are problems with suppositories; many people have psychological objections to them, and they can't always be used when they are needed. "You can't insert a suppository on a bus, but you can swallow a pill without water," remarks one physician tartly. That reasoning accounts for the wide usage of ergotamine in the tablet form.

Generally, the physician will tailor the ergotamine dosage and schedule to each individual patient, experimenting with regimens until the best one is found. That experimentation will include the drugs that are combined with ergotamine. While ergotamine can be taken by itself, drug companies have made available a number of tablets that combine it with such drugs as caffeine, phenobarbital, and phenacetin. The caffeine is added because it also constricts blood vessels, the phenacetin to help kill pain, and the phenobarbital to calm the patient and, hopefully, the queasy stomach. This last point is important, because the vomiting that often accompanies migraine may make it impossible for the patient to keep the tablet down, which means that the drug never gets a chance to do its work. Occasionally, the physician will prescribe a tranquillizer to help calm the patient.

When a physician prescribes ergotamine, he will stay alert for side effects. Generally, patients who follow doctor's orders and report any peculiarities that they notice have little to fear. Caution must also be observed by the physician when treating migraine patients who have heart disease or abnormalities of the blood vessels. Because ergotamine causes blood vessels to constrict, it can worsen these conditions, and should not be used when they are present. And because ergotamine can cause contractions of the womb—at one time ergot was used for that purpose medically—it is not prescribed for pregnant women. However, migraine usually goes away during pregnancy, because of hormonal changes.

In addition to taking ergotamine (and whatever additional drugs the physician prescribes), the migraine patient can take other helpful measures. It's advisable to get into a quiet, dark room, since there is unusual sensitivity to both noise and light during an attack. Lying down, with the head slightly raised, helps ease the pain. A thirsty patient should drink some black coffee, which contains caffeine that helps fight the attack. If vomiting and nausea are severe, antispasmodic drugs that calm down the surging stomach can be taken. For momentary relief, the patient can try pressing on the scalp artery that is causing the trouble. Often, gentle pressure will ease the pain somewhat for a time. So may two tablets of aspirin.

A patient who does all these things usually can count on relief from pain (although other bothersome symptoms of the migraine attack, including nausea, may continue for hours). For most patients, taking enough ergotamine early enough is the key to success. If this isn't done, the headache may continue, changing over a period of hours from a throbbing attack to the dull, steady pain that indicates that the blood vessels have become rigid and pipe-like.

Once that happens, ergotamine is no longer effective against migraine pain, since it can no longer constrict the blood vessels. Now the patient must rely on powerful pain-killing drugs. Except in mild cases, aspirin is not powerful enough to help at this stage, and physicians will prescribe something as strong as morphine or Demerol. Obviously, these are drugs of last resort, and no patient should take them on his own initiative. Morphine and other powerful pain-killers are addictive drugs, and a patient who takes too much of them without careful monitoring by a physician may find himself with a worse problem than migraine: addiction.

Sometimes the physician will try a different approach; he will prescribe a sedative and send the patient to a dark room to literally "sleep it off." Tranquillizers are prescribed less frequently, but some physicians may give them for the same purpose.

For the patient who gets through the migraine attack only to find himself gripped by a muscle contraction headache caused by the tension of having migraine, the route to relief is the same road traveled by all tension headache sufferers: aspirin or other pain-killers, massage, a hot bath or shower, and relaxation. When the attack is finally over, some patients prefer to spend some time in bed, recuperating and enjoying their freedom from pain. It is a tired but happy moment.

But as is the case with tension headaches, getting relief from one migraine attack is just a prelude to a more important effort—to prevent future attacks. In this case, the migraine sufferer is slightly luckier than the tension headache patient, because there is a drug that can be taken by many people to prevent migraine attacks.

The drug, mentioned earlier, is methysergide. When it was introduced in 1959, methysergide appeared to be the answer to the migraine patient's prayers. As is typical with many drugs, however, the dream treatment turned out to have elements of a nightmare, at least for some patients. With continued use, some potentially serious side effects showed up. The most troublesome of these side effects is fibrosis—the formation of clogging fibers in the abdomen, the upper chest, the heart, and around some blood vessels. Sometimes these fibers form so tightly around blood vessels that they clamp down on them, cutting off the blood supply. Methysergide should not be used by people with liver or kidney disease, patients with infections, cardiac patients, and pregnant women. When these conditions do not exist, physicians will still monitor patients closely, to detect any trouble early. Usually, methysergide therapy will be interrupted for at least two or three weeks every six months to minimize the chance of side effects.

Despite all these warnings and precautions, methysergide still remains the most potent drug therapy for preventing migraine attacks. When it is prescribed, most physicians will try to establish the daily dose at the lowest level that will prevent attacks. Some physicians will not use methysergide unless the migraine attacks are frequent and severe. Others will start with a low dose—perhaps one tablet a day—and will increase it only if attacks still occur. (While the dosage is tailored for individual patients, a common recommendation calls for three tablets a day.) Other physicians prefer to start with a high dosage schedule and reduce it as they go along.

Because of methysergide's potent side effects, most physicians now tend to use it as a drug of last resort. In its place, a number of other treatments are being tried.

Many physicians will start by using ergotamine as a preventive drug, often in combination with phenobarbital and an antispasmodic. While ergotamine was not designed for such use, enough physicians have reported good results with it to make it their drug of choice. Instead of waiting for the attack, these physicians find that daily doses of ergotamine can prevent attacks.

If ergotamine does not work, the physician may try cyproheptadine, a drug that neutralizes both serotonin and histamine. If that does not bring relief, a drug named Pizotifen, perhaps better known to physicians by the code name BC 105, may be tried. In some resistant cases, an antidepressant may produce good results. Only if all other alternatives fail will methysergide be tried.

This is an excellent example of how research has enlarged the list of anti-migraine drugs. Cyproheptadine was not developed as a headache drug but to fight allergies; physicians began using it for headache on the theory that any drug which fights the effects of histamine and serotonin could help migraine patients. The same reasoning led to the use of Pizotifen.

Both these drugs have been tested on a large scale in Australia, where researchers report that they are not as successful in as many patients as is methysergide, but that they have fewer side effects. In the United States, there is a paradox of drug therapy caused by our strict drug rules. The Food and Drug Administration, whose job is to protect drug consumers from unnecessary harm, has not officially approved ergotamine or cyproheptadine for use to prevent migraine attacks. Many headache physicians use the drugs for that purpose anyway, despite the FDA's frowns. The important part of this research is not the red tape surrounding the drugs' use but the fact that scientists know enough about the causes of migraine to mount a logical, sustained search for better drugs with some hope of success. This is a lot better than testing drugs at random, an all-too-common practice in drug research.

But few doctors will be satisfied to give a patient drugs and let it go at that. While doctors don't necessarily believe in the "migraine personality," they are absolutely certain that emotional factors play a role in a large number of migraine attacks. As with tension headaches, a number of brief sessions in the physician's office, during which he asks questions about the patient's private life and work, often are essential to treatment of migraine.

But because of migraine's complexity, the questioning won't be as simple as that. As he probes, the physician will be looking for "trigger factors"—anything that can set off a migraine attack. There are an amazingly large number of trigger factors in migraine. Food can do it, and different types of food for different patients; for one it may be chocolate, for another, milk. Sudden weather changes may be the trigger factor for some people. Allergies have been implicated in some cases of migraine—and so the list goes on and on. With women, it is quite common to find migraine linked to the menstrual period; with men, the link is often to the stresses and strains of work. Some patients may have one trigger factor, others may have a number of them.

One common trigger factor is the birth control pill. Headache experts have found a surprising correlation between migraine headaches and the Pill in many women. One physician tells of a fourteen-year-old girl who suffered migraine headaches since the age of eight, at a steady rate of one headache a month. Suddenly she began to have severe migraine attacks almost daily. At first, the physician could find no explanation. Then he discovered that the girl had been taking birth control pills—not for contraception, but because another physician had prescribed them to help the girl's acne. When the pills were discontinued, so were the headaches.

This phenomenon has helped migraine research. It's now known that the hormones in birth control pills can cause blood irregularities that may lead to excessive clotting. Somehow, this effect on the circulatory system is linked to the migraine-type effect that the same hormones have on the circulatory system—another clue for researchers to follow up.

In this welter of confusing factors, the emotions do stand out. For some men, the strain of continued hard work will bring on a migraine attack. Other people will find that migraine comes after a stretch of hard work, just as they are ready to relax and enjoy themselves. Unusual excitement of any kind may set off an attack. Some physicians believe that most migraine attacks can be traced back to suppressed feelings of hostility; the agonies of migraine, they say, are the outlet for emotions that a person will not allow himself (or herself) to express in any other way. And it does seem that many patients with migraine set unusually high goals for themselves and strive for them rigidly, without taking bodily weakness into account. Some experts believe that rigidity of mental outlook is the key—these people will not give way to facts that must be recognized, and the bottled-up emotions must escape somehow; the result is migraine.

It is obvious as researchers look deeper into migraine that no one factor can explain all migraine headaches; there is never going to be a magic cure. Instead, for each patient the physician must painstakingly search out the trigger factors involved. Some patients may have to keep diaries, recording all the events that precede each attack, in order to find the trigger factors. In other cases, the physician may try to induce an artificial migraine attack—for instance, by infusing serotonin or histamine—to confirm a suspicion. Often, the physician will find himself acting as a psychotherapist.

"The prognosis of a patient with migraine should be viewed somewhat as that of a patient with peptic ulcer," wrote Dr. Wolff. "Migraine headache attacks may be terminated, or the interval between episodes greatly prolonged, but unless the subject has discovered a suitable pattern of life and is able to adhere to it, headache will recur." And that, Dr. Wolff noted, means that relief from migraine often is more up to the patient than it is to the physician: "One must appreciate that elimination of the headache may demand more in personal adjustment than the patient is willing to give. It is the role of the physician to bring clearly into focus the cost to the patient of his manner of life. The subject must then decide whether he prefers to keep his headache or attempt to get rid of it."

Because those words were written many years ago, the choice patients face is no longer so stark and direct. If physicians now cannot change their patients' style of life and emotional outlook, they can do much through careful use of drugs to reduce the number of migraine attacks. But drugs carry potentially dangerous side effects with them and are almost never totally effective. For those patients in whom the emotional factors of migraine are paramount, the effort to understand one's self better and to alter patterns of behavior that are harmful is well worth making. And for all migraine patients, the rule of moderation in all things, including the emotions, is a valuable one. Plenty of sleep, a good, balanced diet, avoidance of working too hard and playing too hard, careful preparation for stressful periods—these aren't, strictly speaking, medical measures. But they can do as much as potent drugs to make the lot of the migraine sufferer easier.

For most migraine patients, there is one last word of hope. Migraine usually is not a disease of old age, but of the active years of middle life. In the great majority of cases, migraine attacks begin between the ages of sixteen and thirty-five. At about fifty years of age, they often begin to lessen in frequency and severity, and sometimes they go away completely. In women, the menopause and its change in sex hormone production is an obvious explanation for this observation. Oddly enough, exactly the same thing may be happening in male migraine patients. There is such a thing as the male "menopause," called climacteric, although it rarely is as dramatic as the menopause in women. It's just that the production of male hormones does change in later life, which may have an effect on migraine.

In any event, there is plenty of help available for the migraine sufferer. Some of that help comes in the form of drugs, some of it in the form of advice and better understanding of the emotions. Research promises to produce more and better weapons against migraine. So there is a message for the migraine patient: hang on. Time is on your side.

4.

Cluster Headache

UNTIL A FEW years ago, this type of headache was listed as a form of migraine. While some experts still list it as such, most accept it as a vascular headache that deserves its own separate category, because it differs so markedly from the standard migraine headaches. It goes under a number of names: cluster headache (because the attacks occur in clusters); histamine headache (because histamine seems to be the cause); Horton's syndrome (because it was Dr. Bayard T. Horton of the Mayo Clinic who did the most valuable work on it); and, most imposingly, Horton's histaminic cephalgia, which wraps it up in polysyllables.

Cluster headache attacks are a special breed of cat. Often, the headache begins in the middle of the night, jolting the patient out of bed to set him walking the floor in agony. Whenever it begins, the headache comes on with amazing speed, building to full intensity in only five or ten minutes. "Ask a patient with a cluster headache what it is like and he will tell you the pain is excruciating," says Dr.

Cluster Headache

Perry S. MacNeal of the University of Pennsylvania. "Ask him if he ever hit his thumb with a hammer while he was driving a nail, and he'll say that is just what his headache feels like. Fortunately, the pain only lasts forty-five minutes—seldom over two hours. But during that period the patient is so distraught that he may literally beat his head against the wall."

The word "he" is used with good reason. As migraine headaches tend to be a female phenomenon, cluster headaches tend to be a male malady. One headache expert, Dr. John R. Graham, believes that cluster headache patients are a special type of male, identifiable by their rugged facial appearance, pitted orange skin and easy blushing; these men, Dr. Graham says, tend to be unusually hard-driving in business and at play. He believes that all these factors may be explainable by the effect of personal factors on the body's chemistry, thus producing the cluster headache.

The headache affects only one side of the head, as with migraine. It is often accompanied by sweating, tear-filled eyes and a dripping nose, a flushed face and excessive production of saliva. While the headache is soon gone, the patient can expect more like it—a cluster of headaches over a period of six to eight weeks. After that comes a respite of months, perhaps as long as a year, before the next cluster.

Laboratory work, largely by Dr. Horton, has firmly established the role of histamine in cluster headaches. Histamine is a substance that the body produces to help fight injury, infection or other invasions. Unfortunately, histamine's good effects also cause discomfort; it is histamine that produces the stuffy, running nose of a cold, the unhappy symptoms of hay fever and other allergies, some of the pain of an injury. Because most people know histamine only through taking antihistamine drugs, they tend to think of it as a villain, instead of a useful substance that carries some unfortunate side effects.

But in cluster headaches, histamine is nothing but a

45

villain. In these headaches, a sudden excess production of histamine affects one side of the head. Since one of the effects of histamine is to dilate blood vessels, the result is the brief, violent headache that no patient will ever forget. No one really knows why cluster headaches occur, why they occur in clusters, or why they are so brief. Nevertheless, enough is known for physicians to be able to help many patients.

Because the headache is so short-lived, taking ergotamine does little or no good for a specific attack. Physicians may use injections of other drugs that dilate the blood vessels for relief, but they generally prefer to try to prevent the attacks, on the theory that once one begins, it's too late to do much good.

Methysergide is one standby. Instead of having the patient take it constantly, the physician will try to reserve its use for periods when a cluster of headaches is expected. A daily dosage schedule, tailored to the patient, can prevent the headaches, but not in all cases. Some physicians prefer to use ergotamine, usually in combination with caffeine, as a preventive drug. Sometimes steroid drugs are prescribed along with ergotamine, but physicians tend to be cautious about this because of the potentially serious side effects of steroids.

One form of preventive treatment that requires dedication by both physician and patient is histamine desensitization. The theory behind this, which was first outlined by Dr. Horton, is simple: by giving the patient continued small doses of histamine, the body is allowed to build up a tolerance to the substance, so that it does not react catastrophically to large amounts of histamine. This is essential to the preventive therapy given for hay fever, where small amounts of the substance causing the reaction are injected to help the patient.

Histamine desensitization requires skill on the part of the doctor and patience on the part of the headache sufferer. The patient must come in every day at first, every month eventually, spending about forty-five minutes, during which a histamine solution drips into a vein. The sessions are daily at first and gradually taper off to once a month or so as the months go by. Not every physician will try histamine desensitization, because some who have attempted it have had poor results. One risk, for example, is that giving the patient a shade too much histamine at a session will bring on the very headache that the treatment is supposed to prevent. Some physicians don't think much of the technique, because it has given their patients poor results. But those who have mastered desensitization swear by it. Perhaps the leading American exponent of desensitization is Dr. Robert E. Ryan of St. Louis University Medical School, who has frequently written on the subject.

This difference of opinion is only to be expected. It may surprise patients to know this, but most physicians are aware that a treatment for headache (or any other condition, for that matter) usually is as good as the physician thinks it is. That's because our emotions govern our physical reactions to a surprising degree. If a doctor is unenthusiastic about a treatment, the patient is likely to detect it, and that means the patient is not likely to take the treatment seriously—which means poor results. Says Dr. Perry S. MacNeal of the University of Pennsylvania: "The most potent ingredient in any medication that I give, even if it is a placebo [a sugar pill given to ease a patient's fears], is the enthusiasm with which I administer it."

One therapy that the physician probably will not try in cluster headache is psychotherapy. Unlike the other headaches discussed so far, cluster headache does not seem to have strong ties to the emotions or the personality—although, as with almost all headaches, the way a person feels toward life probably will affect the number and severity of the headaches he has. Both in treating the immediate attack and in preventing future attacks, drugs are the major defense against cluster headaches.

One type of drug that won't be used is the antihistamine. Even though the headache is caused by histamine, physicians have found that antihistamines aren't effective in cluster headaches. Apparently, the problem is that the drug can't get to the point of trouble fast enough and in sufficient quantities. At any rate, there are enough other effective drugs available to insure that most cluster headache patients can get relief from a physician.

If a headache does occur, there are some things that the patient can do. One of the more effective measures is to get out of bed and on his feet. While a migraine patient feels better if he lies down, the cluster headache's pain is worsened by lying down. As for drugs, almost nothing will work fast enough for a short-lived attack, but ergotamine suppositories may help if the headache lasts longer than the usual attack. In general, about all the cluster headache patient can do is pace the floor, and ask his doctor to help prevent future attacks.

5.

Sinus Headache

THE SINUS HEADACHE problem starts with a mystery: no one knows why the sinuses exist. The sinuses are hollows in the bones of the head, and specialists have speculated endlessly about their function. Some say they exist to lighten the bones, others that they once helped sharpen the sense of smell, when survival could depend on that sense; still others that the sinuses add resonance to voice. The one thing everyone agrees on is that the sinuses can cause no end of trouble—and that trouble often leads to headaches. Fortunately, physicians have observed a declining incidence of sinus headache, apparently because modern treatments are more effective against the underlying conditions.

The sinuses that physicians are most concerned with are the nasal sinuses, which are more or less offshoots of the nasal passages. There are four pairs of sinuses, all connected to the nasal cavity either directly or via other sinuses. They are:

The *frontal sinuses*, in the forehead above and behind the eyebrows.

The *maxillary sinuses,* in the cheek bones, on either side of the nose. Physicians sometimes call the maxillary sinus the *antrum*

The *sphenoid sinuses,* behind the upper part of the nose. The *ethmoid sinuses,* between the upper part of the nasal cavity and the lower wall of the eye socket. Unlike the other nasal sinuses, which are open, bone-lined chambers, the ethmoid sinuses are composed of a number of small cells. These are especially vulnerable to infection, because they are centrally located in relation to the other sinuses.

The basic mechanism of all sinus headaches is the same: something blocks the open passages, causing pain. But there is a wide variety of reasons why the passages can become blocked: infection (including the common cold and its complications), allergies (including hay fever and its relatives), tumors, and other growths, and deformations of the nose structure. Each of them can cause long-lasting bouts of headache.

One of the most common causes of sinus headache is the spreading of a nasal infection, such as a cold, to the sinuses. When this occurs, the sinus infection is likely to hang on doggedly, flaring up from time to time. The patient may think that the trouble is caused by a series of colds, when the sinusitis is really to blame.

The particular kind of trouble depends on which sinuses are involved. If the infection is in the maxillary sinuses, there will be an uncomfortable "full" feeling in the cheek over the sinuses. If the frontal sinuses are infected, there will be a severe headache over and behind the eyes, with the pain being aggravated by any movement. Frontal sinus headaches usually begin in the morning, build to a peak, and then gradually fade away before bedtime. Ethmoid sinus infections produce a sense of tightness over the nose, with pain radiating outward to the forehead. The sphenoid sinus is less likely to become infected after colds than are the others.

What happens inside the sinus to cause the trouble is essentially similar to what happens inside the nasal passages during a cold. The mucous membranes lining the sinuses begin to produce thick mucus, which tends to block the passages. This may occur during a cold, when swelling of the nasal mucous membranes and the outpouring of nasal mucous fills up the passages and causes the buildup of pressure. The pain tends to be steady, rather than throbbing, because the pressure is steady.

Anything that contributes to the swelling of the mucous membranes also contributes to the pain. The list of contributing factors includes excitement, cold air, high humidity, emotional reactions, menstruation and many other things. Stooping over, coughing, sneezing, or moving the head violently can add to the pain. Lying down, on the other hand, often helps the sinuses to drain, easing the pain.

Another type of headache occurs not within the sinuses, but just outside of them. When the mucous membranes in the nose swell because of infection, allergy, or another reason, the passages leading to the sinuses may become blocked. Eventually, a semivacuum is created in the blocked sinuses, and that vacuum exerts an inward pull on the sinus wall. The unusual pressure stimulates the pain-feeling nerves, causing an ache.

There are other causes for the same type of results. For example, growths within the sinus can block the passages, causing pain. Such growths generally are not malignant. They include nasal polyps, self-limiting and simple excrescences that are removed with relative ease, and overgrowths of the bone surrounding the sinus. An injury to the head can deform the sinus, possibly producing a continuing headache.

In one sense, treatment of the sinus headache is simple. Since these headaches have a physical cause, rather than being primarily emotional, the physician can cure the headache by eliminating the underlying physical cause. In practice, however, it's often not that simple, for two reasons: many patients don't consult doctors, and sinus trouble is not the easiest complaint for physicians to treat.

On the patient's part, it's easy to blame continuing sinus trouble on a series of colds, rather than on one underlying infection. Since sinus headaches usually are more bothersome than crippling, many busy patients will suffer from one bout to another rather than go to their doctor's office. The kind of self-medication that most people will take often is the kind that the physician will prescribe: aspirin, nose drops, other decongestants. These will give enough temporary relief to keep the patient away from the doctor. The problem, of course, is that means that the headaches will keep coming back.

When the patient does consult the physician, the measures recommended for immediate relief will not be too different: pain-killers, decongestants in one form or another, heat to relieve the pain, a recommendation to lie down when the headache occurs. The next step, eliminating the cause of the headaches, may not be so easy.

For example, most of the symptoms produced by a sinus infection are identical with those produced by an allergy. In fact, many Americans go through life believing that they are cold-prone when they really have an allergy. While some allergies are seasonal, such as hay fever, many others have nothing to do with the seasons; people can be allergic to anything from their own husbands and wives to the living room rug.

If an allergy is causing the problem, the physician must first establish that fact and then track down the cause of the allergy. Usually that means "scratch testing," in which the physician makes a small scratch on the patient's arm and applies whatever substance is suspect. If the arm reddens and swells around the scratch, the culprit has been detected.

Some allergens can be easily avoided; if a patient is allergic to chocolate, milk, or another food, he simple stops eating the food. If it is dog hair or feathers, those can be removed from the home. When the allergens cannot be avoided (as in the case of hay fever or other allergies to pollen), nose drops and antihistamines help relieve the problem. For more permanent relief, a series of desensitizing shots, in which tiny amounts of the allergen are injected over a long period of time, can build up resistance to the allergen. (This is exactly what is done with histamine in the case of cluster headache.)

Infections can often be helped by antibiotics or other drugs. But sometimes the infection settles in and becomes chronic. The maxillary sinus is most prone to chronic infections, the sphenoid sinus is least likely to have a chronic infection. In these cases, several steps beyond the use of drugs may be required to root out the infection.

To diagnose the conditions properly, the physician may order X-rays, or he may try a technique called transillumination, in which he seeks contrasts between the sinuses under powerful lighting; those contrasts will show him exactly where the infection is localized.

For treatment, some specialists will try irrigating the sinus. This simply means squirting a warm saline solution into the troubled sinus, either through the natural opening from the nasal cavity or by perforating the sinus wall. This procedure is used most commonly on the maxillary sinus, because it is easiest to reach. Occasionally, an antibiotic may be introduced during the irrigation, to fight the infection on the spot. When all else fails, minor surgery may be needed to give relief.

To sum up, sinus headaches are among the more difficult to master, both because their cause may not be identified easily and because the sinus condition may be difficult to get at. But diligence on the part of both patient and physician can lead to complete relief for almost every sinus headache sufferer.

6.

Allergic Headache

AN ALLERGY IS an abnormal response of the body's defense system to what should be a harmless element of the environment. It can be compared to a homeowner who is so jittery about burglars that he fires his shotgun at the family dog, blasting a hole in the wall.

There's an added element of truth in that analogy, because the emotions often are involved in allergies, and in the headaches they cause. Physicians can explain in precise terms all the chemical, cellular and nervous system reactions that are produced by an allergy, but they sometimes are at a loss to get at the underlying factors. This doesn't mean that every hay fever sufferer is a candidate for psychotherapy, but it does mean that some short, friendly chats by the physician and the patient often do much to improve the effectiveness of the drugs and other treatment prescribed for the specific allergy.

Recently, Drs. Theodore J. Haywood and John P. McGovern divided all allergic headaches into four different categories, a division accepted by most other experts. These headaches are:

1. Primary allergic headache, in which the allergy itself causes the head pain.

2. Sinus headaches.

3. Pressure referred headache (pain that is caused by pressure on one area of the body, but is felt in another area).

4. Allergic headaches whose primary cause is emotional.

Primary allergic headache occurs in four stages. First the body comes in contact with the allergy-causing substance, which physicians call the allergen. Almost anything can be an allergen for one individual or another; for some unknown reason, the body recognizes this innocuous substance—chocolate, pollen, wool, dog's hair, just to name a few—as an enemy invader. It then begins a well-established defense mechanism to fight off the invasion. An essential part of the system is the release of defense substances such as histamine. It is the annoying side effects of these substances that cause the problem.

In the primary allergic headache, the cause is essentially the same as that of a migraine: the defensive chemicals, such as histamine, cause the blood vessels of the head to dilate, starting a vascular headache. This does not happen to everyone, Drs. Haywood and McGovern report: "One usually does find a positive family history of allergy, a past history of allergic disease, and association of headache with definite concurrent and recurrent allergic symptoms."

The second kind of allergic headache, sinus headache, is discussed at length in Chapter Five.

The third type, pressure referred headache, is similar to some kinds of sinus headache. Instead of the sinus mucous membrane swelling, it is the nasal turbinates (a system of bones in the nose that filter particles from incoming air) that swell, producing pressure and then pain. The pain may be referred—transmitted—to any part of the head, and it may radiate to the neck, shoulders, back, or even into the arms.

The final type of allergic headache is formally called "secondary psychophysiological allergic headache." This is a polite way of saying that people who are tense, depressed and irritable tend to find ways of taking out their problems on themselves. Again, this doesn't mean that every allergy patient is a candidate for the psychiatrist's couch. But it does mean that there can be a large emotional factor in allergy. Researchers have produced all the overpowering symptoms of a major allergic reaction by telling the patient that the allergen was present when it really wasn't. In one experiment, almost half of a group of asthma patients went into classic attacks of allergic asthma when they were given small vials of their particular allergens to sniff. They got dramatic relief by sniffing vials containing effective drugs. In reality, both sets of vials contained nothing but a harmless saline solution.

Obviously, the treatment of the allergy headache whose real basis is emotional will differ from the treatment for a headache whose real cause is an allergic reaction. In practice, the division is not so clearcut as it appears on paper, since emotional problems are an element in almost any kind of headache. Physicians know that a smile or a few minutes of time during which the patient gets undivided attention are a vital part of any treatment for any disease condition.

As far as straight medical treatment goes, the most important part of allergy therapy is to keep the allergen away from the patient. Once the allergen is identified (which may take considerable medical detective work), the patient may have to change his eating habits, get rid of a pet, outlaw certain plants from the house, or stop wearing silk or wool, depending on what allergen is implicated in his case. Perhaps the majority of allergy patients are bothered by pollen; the condition is misnamed hay fever or rose fever, since hay or roses rarely are the plants responsible for the sneezing, itching, steadily running nose that goes with the headache. Unless these sufferers are lucky enough to move to a pollen-free part of the country, they can't get away from the allergen during the sensitive part of the year.

The physician will recommend staying in an air-conditioned room as much as possible, since air conditioning filters out some (but not always all) of the pollen in the air. He will prescribe antihistamines to reduce the trouble. Sensitizing shots can be given over a period of weeks before the pollen season begins. By getting the patient's body used to small doses of allergen, the shots can reduce the bothersome symptoms. In a few especially severe cases, the physician may try steroid hormones for temporary relief, although the potentially severe side effects associated with these hormones make physicians handle them with care. Once a vascular headache begins, ergotamine can help cut the attack short. A mild tranquillizer may be prescribed to raise the pain threshhold, calm the patient generally, and reduce the muscle spasms that can accompany an allergic headache. The physician sometimes will prescribe methysergide as a preventive measure for allergic vascular headaches.

While he prescribes drugs and other therapy, the physician will also take time out to discuss the patient's case more fully. An allergy is seldom as simple as it looks; among the factors that can affect allergic attacks are age, sex, the patient's nutritional state, fatigue, the weather, overexertion, the hormones, and the patient's general emotional balance. By now, it's clear that none of these factors escapes the influence of the others. Emotional condition can swing up and down with changes in the weather; bad news that saddens a person can make pain feel more intense; hard work can either leave a person feeling refreshed or worn out; and so on. All of these factors, working together, can affect the way a patient weathers an allergic attack.

When a physician sits down to talk with an allergy headache patient, his aim is to help the patient understand both the headache and himself better. It may not be possible to remove the allergen from the patient's life, but it may be possible to make a housewife understand that her tendency to worry too much about her son-in-law's business affairs may be responsible for the severity of the headaches that go with her hay fever, or to tell a businessman that a little more time spent relaxing can help cut down on the aspirin and antihistamines he takes.

There is some reason to believe that patients with allergic headaches are born with a body whose systems do not function as smoothly as could be desired. The human body, like most functioning systems, has a certain amount of "play" built into it—that is, it is designed to adjust smoothly to minor changes in the environment. For some people, however, the margin for adjustment is small, so that a relatively tiny change in the weather, in nutritional status, in the chemical composition of body fluids, or in any of the myriad other factors that affect human beings can set off a major adjustment that could lead to a headache. Right now, physicians do not have the kind of detailed tests of the body's regulatory systems that would enable them to pinpoint this sort of condition in a given patient. But they can often recognize the existence of such a condition by the patient's physical and mental reactions to challenges such as an allergy.

No matter how technical or simplified are the terms that the physician uses when he talks to the patient, the message is the same: allergy and the headache that goes with it can be more than just a simple physical problem. It can involve the most basic parts of your life style and your physical makeup. Understanding yourself better can do as much to help your allergic headache as the most powerful drug.

7.

Headaches of the Old

OLDER PEOPLE CAN get just about any headache that troubles younger persons (although migraine blessedly tends to taper off or even fade away with advancing age). But there are a few kinds of headache that are seen predominantly or exclusively in older people. Some of these headaches come along with disease of old age, while others just plague older people for no known reason. Since these are caused by a variety of mechanisms and conditions, the link to advanced years is the only thread that connects them.

Headache of Arthritis

Arthritis ranks with headache both in age—it was described by Hippocrates —and in occurrence. (The big difference is that headache is a symptom and arthritis is a disease.) There are two types of arthritis: rheumatoid arthritis, which can strike at any age and is baffling to physicians in spite of years of research into its cause; and osteoarthritis, a much less serious condition that seems to be caused by simple wear and tear on the body's joints. That makes osteoarthritis and its headache a problem almost exclusively of older people.

The joint is a place where two bones meet. It is a pouch of cartilage, containing the cartilage-lined ends of both bones, which are bathed in fluid that lubricates the constant sliding motion of the bones that occurs whenever a person moves. All in all, a beautiful mechanism.

In arthritis, the mechanism starts to break down. Apparently because of the never-ending wear and tear on the ends of the bones, their cartilage "cushions" start to wear away. Calcium deposits start to build up on the ends of the bones, roughening the formerly smooth area. The roughness produces all the discomforts of osteoarthritis: soreness, pain in the joint, difficulty of movement.

The joints of the neck and the spine are not immune to this gradual process of erosion and roughening. Arthritis in this area can easily cause headache, because the nerves that serve this part of the body also serve the head. Arthritis produces a dull, steady headache that usually starts in the back of the head and spreads upward and forward. Because a person with this kind of headache tends to hold the head rigid, the muscles in the neck will start to tighten up, adding the pain of a muscle contraction headache to the ache of arthritis. The arthritis headache often occurs in the early morning hours, awakening the patient. At first, these headaches occur every few days. But as time goes on, they become more frequent and last longer, sometimes subjecting the patient to almost continual bouts of pain. Anything that brings on an attack of arthritis will bring on such a headache: exposure to drafts, dampness, extreme cold, and occupations like sewing or driving, where the head must he held in a fixed position for long periods.

This kind of headache is common simply because osteoarthritis is so common; it is rare for an oldster to escape at least a touch of arthritis. However, a physician may not be able to diagnose the cause of the headache in cases where the presence of arthritis is obvious. Examination of other joints can help prove the case; often, the physician will X-ray the neck and upper spine to detect the characteristic bone changes that are caused by osteoarthritis.

Controlling the arthritis headache means controlling arthritis, a feat that medical science still has not mastered. Millions of dollars are spent annually by naive arthritis patients in search of a cure for their ailment. But in spite of all the fantastic claims made by quacks, there is no cure for arthritis. The most that doctors can do is to slow down the course of the disease and provide a measure of relief from its pain and discomforts—which is, of course, quite enough for many a patient who has been suffering the misery of arthritis.

Generally, the preferred treatment for arthritis is the simplest kind of therapy. In drugs, the standby is aspirin, or other members of the salicylate family to which aspirin belongs. In spite of all the new drugs discovered in recent years, the combination of aspirin's good pain-killing ability and low level of adverse side effects make it the drug of choice for arthritis, and for headaches caused by arthritis. Only if aspirin bothers a particular patient, or if it does not give the required relief, will the physician turn to other drugs whose potency is tempered by the possibility of harmful side effects. A variety of these drugs is available. The most powerful are the steroid hormones, which also have the most powerful side effects. Still, for the patient with intractable pain from arthritis, the risk of side effects may be well worth taking for a respite from pain.

Aside from drugs, other measures can help reduce the pain. Bed rest is one of them. Aside from taking the strain off the spine, bed rest also permits the patient to fight fatigue, which makes the pain feel worse. Heat treatments, ranging from a hot water bottle to hot baths to an infrared lamp, can provide major help; in some cases, massage and carefully designed exercises will be prescribed by the physician. Both massage and exercise obviously should be undertaken with caution, since they can make matters worse if they are mishandled.

In general, the doctor will do whatever he can to keep the patient's physical and mental condition as good as possible, since this will enable the patient to meet the challenge of arthritis better. This may mean dietary recommendations, vitamins, perhaps even advice to move to a better climate, if that is feasible. Lolling in the sun, eating well and getting plenty of sleep and healthy moderate exercise may not eliminate arthritis and its headaches, but they do make them easier to endure.

Headache of Glaucoma

The headache caused by the eye disease called glaucoma can be severe, but it may be the most welcome pain in the patient's life. That's because it can give the warning needed to save his sight. Ignored, glaucoma can slowly but steadily squeeze vision out of existence. Properly treated, it will do little or no damage in most cases. The treatment is simple, usually no more than daily use of eye drops. But detecting the disease may not be so easy—except when the excruciating pain that it creates sends the patient to a doctor.

To understand glaucoma, it's necessary to understand the anatomy of the eye. Very roughly, the eye is a ball filled with a transparent, jellylike substance called the vitreous humor. In the front of the ball is a double-paned window: on the outside the transparent cornea, on the inside the iris that gives the eye its color. In the back of the ball is the retina, which receives images and sends them on to the brain for interpretation through the optic nerve, whose ending can be seen as a flat white disc in the middle of the retina.

In between the cornea and the iris there is a flowing supply of lubricant, the aqueous humor. In the normal eye, the aqueous humor flows away as fast as it is secreted by small glands in the eye. In glaucoma, something goes wrong with the disposal system, and the fluid begins to accumulate. As it does, pressure builds up in the eyeball. When the pressure gets too high, it begins to injure the optic nerve. Left unchecked, the fluid buildup caused by glaucoma can result in blindness—and the disease is one of the leading causes of blindness among older people in the United States.

Glaucoma usually does not begin until age forty-five or so. It can be insidious. The visual symptoms include brief episodes of blurred vision, difficulty in seeing in the dark, and, most important, the appearance of colored halos around strong lights. Loss of vision, when it begins, usually starts on the periphery, and it can be so gradual that the patient doesn't realize what's happening.

The headaches of glaucoma can be equally subtle and insidious. They generally are concentrated in the area of the affected eye. Often, there is an uncomfortable feeling of pressure within the eye. In the early stages of the disease, the headaches can come on at any time. The pain is steady, not throbbing, and it tends to last.

Sometimes, however, a glaucoma headache comes on with sudden, severe intensity; the eye becomes inflamed and nausea and vomiting often accompany the head pain. Curiously, this kind of intense attack is better for the patient in the long run, since it will drive almost anyone to the doctor for relief. Once at the doctor's office, most cases of glaucoma are easy to detect and treat.

Using an instrument called a tonometer, the physician will test for a pressure buildup in the eyeball. He looks for a cloudy, "streamy" cornea, a pupil that is fixed and dilated, and for losses in vision. The signs of glaucoma are unmistakeable in most cases.

Treatment usually means eyedrops—often miotics, which prevent damage to the eye, or a drug to decrease fluid formation. In most cases, diligent use of the eyedrops will prevent further damage. But if the eyedrops do not work, the physician may recommend surgery to improve the eye's drainage system.

One way or another, physicians can handle most cases of glaucoma, once the patient comes to them. That's why it is vital for anyone with a steady headache concentrated around the eye to get to a doctor at once. Once damaged, the optic nerve never recovers. Quick treatment for glaucoma can not only prevent headache, it can also make the difference between sight and blindness.

Temporal Arteritis

While it is not always as dangerous as the headache of glaucoma, temporal artery headache (temporal arteritis) also demands immediate attention, because it can cause partial or even complete loss of vision if left untreated. As is the case with glaucoma, the cause of the condition is unknown; for some reason, the lining of the temporal arteries (which run vertically up the head just in front of the ear, with smaller branches leading away) becomes thicker and stiffer, usually after age sixty. Other arteries of the head may also be affected, but the change is most noticeable in the temporal artery, which can be seen throbbing during an attack.

The headache of temporal arteritis may affect one or both sides of the head. It is intense, throbbing and persistent, usually with a burning feeling that is felt in few other headaches. The temporal arteries often are painful to the touch, and chewing may be painful.

Aside from the headache, the patient may suffer from loss of vision, partial or total, which lasts only for a short while. Nausea, vomiting, loss of appetite and weight loss often go along with the visual symptoms and the headache; fever, weakness, and a general weak feeling occur in some cases. The headaches usually build in severity as time goes on, lasting for hours at a time. But often, it is visual trouble instead of the headache that brings the patient to the doctor. That's because aspirin or other painkillers can give enough headache relief to keep the patient comfortable, so that medical attention does not seem necessary. But few people can ignore serious trouble with their vision, and they rush to have their eyes looked at. That may make the diagnosis difficult at first, but the key sign—the throbbing temporal artery—usually tells the story to the alert physician.

For immediate pain relief, the physician may give an injection of local anesthetic, such as procaine, in the area of the artery. For more lasting relief, he usually will prescribe one or another of the steroid hormones, which reduce the swelling of the arteries and improve blood flow; as a result, the headache and other symptoms will disappear. When the steroids do not work, minor surgery may do the job. This is a relative simple operation, often performed under local anesthetic because the temporal artery is so easy to get at. The surgeon opens the skin and ties off the artery, cutting off both the flow of blood and the pain. The whole procedure requires only a few days in the hospital. Tying off the artery usually does no harm, because the body adjusts by sending the blood through alternate arteries that serve the same general area.

As effective as the treatment is, the headache must be treated to do the patient any good. Physicians warn that any unexplained severe headache in an elderly person calls for quick attention. The temporary loss of vision that accompanies temporal arteritis can become permanent in some cases without the proper treatment. Once again, this is a headache that the patient ignores at his own risk.

Meniere's Syndrome

Although most people do not realize it, the ear is for more than just hearing. Within the inner ear is a structure called the labyrinth, whose function is to allow us to keep our balance. You can upset the labyrinth temporarily by spinning rapidly to produce dizziness. In the condition called Meniere's syndrome, nature does something to interfere .with the functioning of the labyrinth. The result is dizziness, a loss of hearing, tinnitus (ringing in the ear)—and headache.

65

Meniere's syndrome usually does not strike until the age of forty-five or later. It takes the form of recurring attacks, during which the patient becomes disoriented, dizzy, hears ringing noises and suffers from headache. The attacks and the headaches that go with them become worse; sometimes the headaches continue after the attack ends. Usually, only one ear is affected by the condition.

There are two types of headache in Meniere's syndrome. One is a one-sided pain on the affected side of the head, usually throbbing but sometimes taking the form of a steady pain. A second variety is a sustained feeling of tightness, pressure and ache all over the back of the head and neck.

As is the case with other headaches caused by organic conditions, the right way to treat the headache is to treat the condition. Unhappily, Meniere's syndrome is one condition that medical science has not been able to cope with very successfully. A wide variety of drugs is used—one sign that none of the drugs is particularly effective. One ultramodern technique uses high-frequency sound waves to inactivate the labyrinth while leaving the hearing unaffected. In many cases, the condition simply runs its course. In these cases, the deafness becomes permanent—which means that the ringing in the ear ends—but the dizziness often persists. Generally, the headaches will stop when the condition is far advanced. Until then, aspirin or other pain-killers are used to relieve the headaches. Medical researchers are working toward better methods of treating this baffling condition.

Basilar Artery Insufficiency

The basilar artery is at the base of the brain—clearly, a crucial location. When its blood flow capacity is lessened, which often happens during old age because of the general stiffening and thickening of artery walls that comes with advancing years, a number of disturbances, including headaches, can result. They include visual disturbances, dizziness, paralysis, and numbness of one side of the head.

The headache that goes with this condition usually is intense, throbbing, and long-lasting. It can be aggravated by changes of posture.

Apparently, what happens is that the arteries on the exterior of the skull dilate so they can supply the blood that the basilar artery cannot carry. When the dilation goes too far, a vascular headache begins. Since the shortage of blood flow in the basilar artery is more or less permanent, the headache is likely to continue for long periods. The other symptoms are due to shortages of blood suffered by parts of the brain that control specific functions. They vary according to the site where blood flow is interfered with and the efficiency with which other arteries make up the deficiency.

Treatment of the condition often involves drugs that can increase the flow of blood through the constricted artery. Because of the throbbing nature of the pain, this headache can be confused with migraine. Detailed physical and laboratory tests, including X-rays, may be necessary for the physician to make the proper diagnosis and prescribe the correct treatment.

□ □ □

These are by no means all the headaches that can affect the elderly. Older persons can suffer from virtually any type of headache that affects their juniors, from sinus headache to migraine. However, some types of pain are found most often in the elderly, either because of known physical changes that come with aging or for reasons that medical science still cannot grasp.

As can be seen, the headaches peculiar to old age are a decidedly mixed bag, with no physical cause in common. If they do have anything in common, it is the possibility of increased damage unless they are given skilled medical treatment. You can live with migraine or tension headache by adjusting to the pain, but you can't live with glaucoma or temporal arteritis without the real risk of blindness. That's not the kind of risk that anyone, of any age, would want to take. Unfortunately, many older people make a point of not seeing the doctor about many complaints, often because they think they can't afford it. Medicare helps fight that belief, but there's an even stronger argument, one that was mentioned earlier: a headache is a symptom of something wrong. Especially for older people, the worst thing to do is to ignore the underlying condition that causes the headache while seeking temporary relief among the nostrums that line the druggist's shelves. At any age, the gift of sight is too valuable to lose for any reason—especially a financial reason. That's why any of the headaches described above is cause for seeing the family physician, without wasting time on self-medication.

8.

Headaches of the Young

YES, CHILDREN DO get headaches—the full range and variety of headaches that their parents get, although, fortunately, not as many of them. Childhood is usually a happy time, free of the tensions that come with adult responsibilities, and free of the headaches that those responsibilities so often produce.

In diagnosing children's headaches, physicians use essentially the same principles that they do in adult cases—with one notable difference. If it is a case of migraine, the physician will look for a family history, trigger factors such as certain foods, and the emotional characteristics that are typical of migraine headaches. If it is a tension headache, the physician will look for factors at school or at play that are disturbing the child. He will also look for physical factors, such as eyestrain, diseases and epilepsy, that could be responsible for headaches.

But in almost every case, the physician will also be interested in the parents of the child with a headache. Children normally learn by imitating, and they may learn quickly that complaining about a headache the way that mommy does is an excellent way to get out of doing chores or completing a homework assignment. Or headaches may be a child's way of reacting to an unpleasant home situation. It's natural for the physician to focus on the parents, because they play such a major role in the child's emotional life, and emotional life plays a predominant role in headaches at any age.

On the other hand, parents shouldn't be quick to blame themselves for a child's headaches. Children are quite different from adults, in their physical needs as well as their mental activities. A child's headache, like the brief, violent fevers that so often go with minor childhood diseases, may be no more than an indication of the special physical characteristics of the early, growing years. Or it may be that both physical and emotional factors, inside the home and outside, too, are all involved in the headaches. In short, diagnosing a child's headache is as big a challenge as any adult headache diagnosis offers.

Migraine

Migraine in children is more common than many parents realize. Any parent with a family history of migraine should be on the alert for it to show up. It can start surprisingly early, often under age ten in boys. Girls, for some reason, tend to develop migraine only after age twelve.

The symptoms of migraine in children can be quite different from the adult experience. For one thing, the gastrointestinal symptoms—nausea and vomiting—are much more prominent in children. They may be so much more alarming than the headache that physicians may diagnose the condition as a gastrointestinal disorder instead of migraine. In some cases, the symptoms are much more confusing. A mother may bring her young son to the doctor's office complaining that he has brief periods during which he seems unusually confused and agitated, with alarming indications that his thinking is unclear. In her agitation about these disturbing symptoms, the mother may not notice the headache that accompanies them, and the physician may diagnose the child as having a psychosis or a convulsive disorder, such as epilepsy.

In saying this, he may not be far from wrong. There is a vague but definite link between epilepsy and migraine. Electroencephalograms often show unusual brain waves in migraine patients that are reminiscent of epilepsy. Some studies indicate that epilepsy and migraine go together more often than pure chance might indicate. No one suggests that migraine leads to epilepsy or vice versa, but the relationship between the two conditions intrigues investigators. The fact that migraine in children can be mistaken for a kind of epilepsy adds to the interest that some researchers have in exploring the link.

Difficulty in making the proper diagnosis diminishes as the child gets older, since the pattern tends to change to typical adult migraine attacks in which the one-sided, throbbing headache is the most prominent factor. However, the juvenile type of migraine, with its contradictory symptoms, may persist into the teens.

Treatment of migraine in children is much the same as treatment in adults. Methysergide may be used to prevent attacks, but many physicians shy from giving such a potent drug to children. Some physicians have reported the successful use of ergotamine to prevent attacks; others will use a common tranquillizer such as phenobarbital. Because depression is very common with childhood migraine, the physician may also prescribe drugs to treat this condition.

The doctor may also want to discuss the family atmosphere with the parents, if only because no one is sure how much of childhood headache is purely hereditary and how much is caused by the specific incidents of family life. If one or both parents suffer from migraine, the physician may recommend talking less about it while the child is present. A child who is brought up in a home where the parents discuss headaches constantly is more likely to complain of headaches himself than one who comes from a headache-free home.

In treating the migraine attacks, the physician runs into a major difficulty: because nausea and vomiting are so predominant, the child may not be able to keep down ergotamine tablets. In addition, most children are reluctant to use suppositories, no matter how effective they are. Inhalation of ergotamine often is prescribed, although the inhalation device is not easy for a child to use. The other drugs used to treat childhood migraine are similar to those used for the adult condition.

Tension Headaches

Tension headaches in children, as in adults, are caused by pressure and stress. Children, naturally, are under different pressures than are their parents, but the results are the same. And as is the case with adults, many tension headaches in children have depression as their root cause.

Take Susan R., an unusually bright eight-year-old whose parents were striving, ambitious, and very proud of their daughter's school record. Thanks to her high grades—due in large part to coaching by the parents—Susan was jumped ahead to a class of ten-year-olds. Intellectually, she found no difficulty in keeping up with the work. But socially, she found herself in a strange world where everyone was bigger, where she could not break into the closed groups of friends, and where she often found herself sitting alone and neglected at lunch and recess. In a few weeks, Susan's headaches began—first on Sundays, in anticipation of the approaching school week, then almost every night as her loneliness and anxiety increased. Her headaches did not end until the family physician diagnosed their cause, held a long talk with the parents, and wrote a letter to the school recommending that Susan be transferred to a class of children her own age.

"Tension headaches in children are nearly always due

to school pressures," says Dr. Harry H. Garnet of the Chicago Medical School. "The kids are pushed, they are skipped ahead in their school work, they are under great obligations to succeed—particularly the advanced student. It's the one who doesn't give a damn who never has headaches."

There are, of course, other causes of children's tension headaches—the anxieties of approaching puberty, teasing by other children, a strained family life. To treat these headaches, the physician may prescribe a tranquillizer or aspirin as a temporary measure. But his major effort will be to the cause of the tension. Often, that will require the same kind of psychotherapy needed to investigate the causes of adult tension headaches, except that both parents and the child will be included in these sessions. It may require a good deal of patience to get at the root of the problem, but the effort is needed. Pain-killers may make the child comfortable for a time, but nothing but an end to the abnormal life situation can eliminate the tension headaches.

Other Childhood Headaches

Eyestrain is a frequent cause of headaches in children. The symptoms are fairly clear-cut: complaints about eyestrain or discomfort during the morning in class, followed by a headache that ebbs during lunch, when the child can rest his eyes, but returns in the afternoon. An eye examination, often ending with the prescription of glasses to correct a visual problem, is vital in these cases.

The sinus problems, colds, and allergies that cause headaches in adults can often cause them in children; in these cases, treatment is almost exactly the same as for adults. An added cause of childhood headaches is the occurrence of measles, mumps, or another of the common diseases of children. These headaches usually signal the onset of the disease, and go away after the first hours or days. Otitis media—infection of the inner ear—often is accompanied by a sharp, feverish headache. Treatment of the underlying infection is important in otitis media to prevent the infection from spreading to the mastoids, where it can cause much more trouble.

Once upon a time, not too long ago, parents were told to be alert for a sudden summer headache, because it could be the first warning sign of paralytic polio. That headache, thankfully, is no longer a threat. The Salk and Sabin vaccines have removed the specter of infantile paralysis that once hung over every American child.

9.
High Blood Pressure and Headaches

In the past two decades, high blood pressure has become one of the major health preoccupations of the American people. That's hardly surprising, because high blood pressure has been linked directly to heart disease and other ailments of the vascular system, and these ailments cause half of all the deaths in the United States. American men, especially, have been changing their diet, exercising, and giving up cigarettes—at least temporarily—because of the statistics linking hypertension (the medical name for high blood pressure; it's a word that literally means "high pressure") and sudden death from heart attack, stroke, and other diseases of the cardiovascular system.

Those statistics are definite: the higher the blood pressure, the greater the chance of having a heart attack. (Add cigarette smoking, no exercise and a high-fat diet, and the chances of having a heart attack skyrocket.) The statistics linking hypertension and headache aren't there, at least not in any great number. Nevertheless, most people with hypertension, and a good number of physicians, are convinced that the hypertension headache exists. Most of them describe it in the same way: a dull ache in no particular part of the head that usually starts in the morning and fades away by the afternoon. The pain may be minor, or it may be intense. In some cases, it goes on and on, rather than ending after a few hours.

Despite this firm description, a number of doctors have been sceptical about the link between hypertension and headache. They reason that most middle-aged American men suffer from hypertension to some degree, but that the people who tend to show up in doctor's offices to have their blood pressure taken are nervous types, acutely aware of every symptom, whose nervousness makes them more prone to tension headaches. These doctors don't doubt that men with hypertension have headaches. They just doubt that the hypertension causes the headaches.

That doubt seems to have been disproved by a recent medical study made by a team of physicians in Scotland. In the most impeccable manner of conducting research, the investigators took two groups of patients. One group consisted of persons with hypertension; within the group, the degree of hypertension ranged from mild to severe. The second group was made up of persons with normal blood pressure, who were matched as carefully as possible in every other respect—age, income, etc.—with the hypertensive group. Once they had made the match, the investigators asked members of both groups about their headaches.

They found that persons with mild or moderate hypertension had just about the same number of headaches experienced by persons in the matched group with normal blood pressure. But for persons with severe hypertension, the picture was different. These people had more headaches than the group with normal blood pressure—and the greater the hypertension, the greater the occurrence of headaches. What's more, the headaches described by persons with severe hypertension fit the standard description of the hypertension headache almost exactly—starting in the morning, vanishing by noon, and so on. The investigators also found that the headaches diminished when the hypertension was brought under control by following a physician's instructions.

That study seems to clinch the case: the hypertension headache does exist. It's logical that it should. In hypertension, the pressure on the blood vessel walls is increased. And as already noted, dilation of blood vessels is a leading cause of headache. In its own way, the hypertension is a vascular headache.

But a full understanding of hypertension and the headache it can cause requires a brief sketch of that everyday miracle, the cardiovascular system—that is, the heart and the vessels through which it pumps blood. We accept the working of this system as routine, because each of us has one. It might help achieve a proper appreciation to point out that the best efforts of all our scientists and engineers have not been able to duplicate the system's silent, efficient operation for more than a few hours, compared to the decades that the typical heart works without complaint.

But the heart does not do its work alone. With every heartbeat, blood is pumped out into the arteries. Under the pressure of the oncoming blood, the arteries expand somewhat. As they contract again, they force the blood ahead through a series of natural valves that keep the blood flowing in the right direction. When the arteries are completely contracted, another heartbeat starts the cycle again.

So there are two moments in time at which the pressure within the arteries can be measured: the moment when the heart contracts, expanding the arteries, and the moment just before the heartbeat, when the arteries are fully contracted. The first moment measures the *systolic* pressure—blood pressure at its highest point. The second moment, the moment of *diastolic* pressure, measures blood pressure at its lowest point. Customarily, physicians list systolic pressure first: a listing of "140 over 80" means a systolic blood pressure of 140 and diastolic pressure of 80.

No one is born with a given blood pressure that remains constant for a lifetime. Newborn infants have systolic pressures under 60, but that soon begins to climb. Blood pressure increases gradually until the teens. Then, normally, it levels off, climbing slowly through the years of maturity.

That's what should happen. Too often in our society it doesn't. It is quite common for American men to have hypertension, as the heart attack statistics testify. The effort to cut the American death rate has set off a major research effort aimed at discovering the causes of hypertension and its link with heart disease. That effort has been at least partially successful. Among the factors linked to hypertension and heart disease have been a fat-rich diet, which tends to cause accumulation of fatty deposits in the arteries, making them stiffer and narrower and thus raising pressure; tension, anger and other disturbing emotions, which seem to affect blood pressure by acting on the nervous system; cigarette smoking, apparently because chemicals in the smoke constrict the vessels; and excess salt consumption, which causes an increase in fluid content, driving up pressure within the arteries. But there are also many cases in which blood pressure is abnormally high for no visible reason. Whatever the reason, the average American blood pressure is likely to be above the level that physicians regard as desirable.

In addition to headache, there are other symptoms of hypertension—dizziness, weakness, numbness of the hands or feet and light-headedness. Needless to say, the emotions play a part in most of these symptoms, including headache; studies have shown that blood pressure can zoom up or down in a matter of minutes in response to such innocuous stimuli as a visit to the doctor's office. This tendency for nervousness and hypertension to go together muddies the headache picture somewhat. A nervous, hypertense person who develops a tension headache tends to blame it all on the hypertension, but studies indicate that the headaches can occur even when the blood pressure is lower than usual for the patient. The best way to sum it up is to say that hypertension and the emotions are so intertwined that no clear line can be drawn between purely tension headaches and purely hypertensive headaches in persons suffering from high blood pressure.

Treatment for hypertension headaches does include the kind of informal psychotherapy that doctors employ for any other kind of headache. But the keystone of the treatment will be the effort to relieve the underlying condition. Over the years, research has produced a wide variety of drugs aimed at hypertension, and they will be an important element of the treatment. The most widely employed of these drugs are diuretics, which remove fluid from the body. Millions of persons with hypertension now take daily doses of diuretics, usually supplementing the activity of the drugs with low-salt diets. Another family of drugs for hypertension operates on a completely different principle. These drugs act on the nervous system to keep blood vessels from constricting unduly, thus keeping blood pressure within more normal limits.

In addition to drugs, the physician will have a number of recommendations for the patient with hypertension. They include losing weight, since extra pounds add to the work that the heart must perform; giving up cigarette smoking, which can be recommended to anyone for any condition; getting more sleep; and eating sensibly—not only watching cholesterol and other fats, but also avoiding heavy meals in general.

Exercise is a touchier subject. In principle, every American man and women should be leading an active, athletic life. In practice, most people today are so badly out of shape that they run the risk of doing themselves serious harm unless they are very careful about their exercise. The middle-aged man who gets up from his armchair and decides to recapture his youthful figure by jogging can jog himself right into a heart attack unless he takes some precautions: he should first see a doctor to have his medical condition checked, then carefully plan a program that will build up his endurance slowly. Exercise is great. It can help you lose weight, sleep sounder, feel better and live longer. It can provide a release for tensions that is more effective than tons of aspirin for headache relief. But for anyone in a sedentary job who hasn't done hard physical work for years, exercise can be a killer, unless it's handled right. Paperback manuals on the latest fad in exercising aren't enough. It's best to see the family doctor before undertaking any intensive program of exercise.

If these measures fail to work in runaway cases of hypertension, surgery may be tried as a drastic measure. In the operation, the surgeon will cut the nerves which run to the blood vessels of the abdominal area, a step that often causes blood pressure to fall. But the operation requires a long period of hospitalization and does not always work, so it is reserved for serious cases.

For most people, good sense and moderation can take the place of such drastic measures as surgery. Relaxation, a good night's sleep, sensible eating habits, moderate but regular exercise, avoiding cigarettes and trying to remain serene amidst the trials of life are wise ways to avoid hypertension with its headaches and other troubles.

10.

Headache and the Eyes

MOST PEOPLE ARE likely to blame their eyes for many tension headaches. In fact, difficulties with vision do not rank that high on the list of causes for chronic headaches. When visual problems are at fault, the headaches often are relatively easy to treat. But it's easy to see why eyes often get the blame. Man is essentially a seeing animal, getting the great majority of his information about the world through his eyes, and so people are acutely aware of the possibility of eye trouble. Because of that, it's often easier to say that eyestrain causes chronic headaches than to admit that personal problems are behind recurrent bouts of tension headaches.

Nevertheless, the eyes can be responsible for headaches. One particularly serious type of headache caused by eye trouble is the headache of glaucoma, discussed in Chapter Seven, which requires immediate attention by a physician. Glaucoma's headache is relatively easy to detect, since the pain is concentrated around the eye.

81

Other types of headaches caused by less serious eye problems are not nearly as localized, and so may require more testing before the cause can be established.

The eye is a device for receiving light waves and transforming them into information that can be interpreted by the brain. The essence of the eye's functioning is the delicate mechanisms that are set up to insure that the light waves are received properly. Each eye has six muscles, in three pairs, which pull the eyeball into position. The eye's lens must then focus the light waves precisely on the retina, where the information is transmitted to the brain. Both eyes must work in close coordination to avoid double vision. When anything goes wrong with any one of these systems, eyestrain and headache can result.

Perhaps the muscles are not coordinated properly. That lack of coordination can cause squinting and unusual strain of the muscles, which often leads to a typical back-of-the-head tension headache.

Perhaps something is wrong inside the eye, so that the incoming light waves are not focused properly on the retina. If the image focuses in front of the retina, nearby objects are seen clearly, but everything in the distance is a blur; the condition is called myopia, or nearsightedness. If the image comes to a focus behind the retina, nearby objects are blurred, but far-off scenes are clear, in what physicians call hyperopia and laymen call farsightedness. In our society, myopia is much more common than hyperopia, apparently because of all the close-up work and reading required of children and adults alike. An additional problem that affects adults more than children is astigmatism, which is caused by irregular curvature of the light-focusing mechanism. Astigmatism can occur with either myopia or hyperopia. In old age, eye trouble may be caused by presbyopia, gradual hardening of the lens that makes it more difficult for the eye to focus. Presbyopia, which usually starts in the forties, is the major reason why older people tend to start holding newspapers or books at arm's length.

Headache and the Eyes

Any of these visual difficulties can cause eyestrain. As the person struggles to achieve normal vision with abnormal eyes, he is literally straining his eyes. Vision may become blurred, the eyes may redden; rubbing them constantly worsens the reddening and makes them water. As the struggle goes on, headache begins—essentially a tension headache, starting at the back of the neck and working upward, but sometimes concentrated in the area of the eyes. Usually, the pain is steady and persistent, but it can imitate the throb of migraine.

Generally, eyestrain headache will not occur until the day is well under way, because it takes some time for eyestrain to make itself felt. Resting the eyes often brings temporary relief, but the pain comes back when the struggle to see resumes. That should make the diagnosis simple, except for the fact that some eyestrain headaches can occur when there's nothing wrong with the eyes. Bad lighting conditions, awkward seating arrangement, and similar circumstances that make seeing difficult can also cause eyestrain and headache.

This all sounds horrendous, but for most people the danger isn't too great. The majority of Americans take better care of their eyes than they do of the rest of their bodies. Schools routinely check vision every year, and anxious mothers complete the job by bringing their children to the ophthalmologist for regular check-ups. A couple of decades ago, teachers were much less conscious of eye problems, and it was rare to see a child wearing eyeglasses. Today, young eyes get careful attention and it's common to see even four-year-olds wearing eyeglasses. We might even overdo it, but that's better than discovering the need for eyeglasses only after persistent headaches drive the mother to the family doctor for help.

Eyestrain headache is more common among adults, because they often don't recognize the fact that the eyeglasses that were prescribed a decade ago are no longer satisfactory. The eyes do change with age, but several factors, including the ego ("There's nothing wrong with *my* eyes!'') and the gradualness of the change can produce eyestrain.

Fortunately, the eyestrain and headache are eliminated with relative ease in most cases. As a matter of routine, physicians will test the eyes of any patient with chronic headaches. If there is something wrong, eyeglasses—or a new prescription for outdated glasses—usually will put things right again. The situation is more complicated when bad lighting or other external factors cause the eyestrain. Some medical detective work may be required to track down the culprit. But once the cause is established, the solution of the problem is simple: a brighter light bulb, a better chair to make reading and writing easier, a lamp that gives less glare can do away with eyestrain and headache almost overnight.

11.
Brain Diseases and Headaches

IF AMERICANS ARE sensitive to the possibility of eye trouble causing headaches, they are terrified at the possibility that their headaches might be caused by a disease of the brain. No one really knows how many headache sufferers stay away from doctors out of fear of being told that a brain tumor or some other frightening condition is responsible, but the number probably is large. That's bad for two reasons: in the vast majority of cases, those fears are completely unfounded and the patient is not getting the relief from pain that a physician could provide. In the small number of patients who do have a disturbance of the brain causing headaches, quick medical attention usually is vital if the problem is to be overcome. But just to emphasize the point again, fears that brain tumors cause recurring headaches are totally erroneous in all but a very few cases.

In fact, one rule that physicians use to eliminate brain diseases as a cause of headache is a long history of headache in an individual. "When a patient comes in and tells me she's had headaches every week for twenty years, with indigestion and problems like that, I'm likely to feel better about it," says one physician. "It means that I don't have to worry about a serious organic disease."

Nevertheless, these organic diseases do happen. Anyone who is afraid of such a disease should go see a doctor at once. The odds are that the physician, after a physical examination, will be able to reassure the patient that no organic disease is present, allowing both doctor and patient to start working toward headache relief.

Brain Tumor

There may be two more frightening words in the language than these, but these will do to scare most people. In actuality, however, the condition may not be bad as most people believe. There are two types of brain tumor, benign and malignant. A benign tumor grows slowly and does not spread to other parts of the body. Once removed, a benign tumor is no longer a cause for worry. A malignant tumor, on the other hand, tends to grow more rapidly, and it can send colonies of cancerous cells to other parts of the body, where they take root and grow. Even if the main tumor is removed, these distant colonies pose a severe danger. Both rapid growth and the tendency to metastisize—spread to other parts of the body—make malignant tumors highly dangerous.

The symptoms of both types of tumor are the same. As they grow, tumors exert pressure on the brain, interfering with its functions. Hearing, sight or speech may be impaired, or partial paralysis may occur. But one of the leading symptoms of brain tumor is headache—a deep, steady aching headache that appears with little warning and is made worse by coughing, sneezing or changes of posture. Aspirin or other pain-killers may relieve the pain at first, but the increasing pressure of the enlarging tumor causes a recurrence. As the tumor grows, pressing more heavily on the brain, both the headache and other symptoms worsen; the patient may suffer loss of memory or even a change of personality.

The answer to brain tumor is removal of the tumor. In many cases, radiation treatment will precede surgery. The radiation is used to kill as much of the tumor as possible, so that removal is easier. In some cases, radiation alone will be used, but surgical removal of the tumor is the usual course of action.

For those who worry overly about brain tumor, it should be stressed that recurring headaches are no definite indication of a tumor; indeed, many brain tumors produce no headache at all. And again, it must be stressed that merely worrying about the possibility of having a brain tumor does no one any good. Whether or not the worry is groundless, a visit to the family physician is definitely advisable.

Brain Abscess

An abscess is a pocket of infection where bacteria, fluid and damaged tissue accumulate, forming a little packet of trouble. In the brain, an abscess often produces the same kind of symptoms as a tumor—imparied hearing, speech, vision or other bodily functions, partial paralysis, loss of memory—for the same reason: the accumulated material in the abscess is disturbing the brain by pressure. But an abscess will also produce a high fever, which is absent in a brain tumor.

The headache produced by a brain abscess sometimes is felt at the site of the abscess, but sometimes can be remote from that spot. In other respects it is like the headache caused by a tumor: steady, often aching, aggravated by coughing and other straining activities.

Brain abcesses have a variety of causes. Perhaps the most common is an infection of the middle ear that spreads until it reaches the brain. Sinus infections that spread to the brain are another common cause of abscesses. ("Common" is a relative word; fortunately, the widespread use of antibiotics against infections has greatly lessened the serious nature of these conditions and the occurrence of brain abscesses.) Injuries to the head can also cause abscesses; when a bruised scalp becomes infected, or when a piece of bone is driven into the brain, for example. Some abscesses have immediate, acute effects, while others may smoulder for years, causing recurrent headaches and the disturbing symptoms that accompany them.

Antibiotics often are used to treat brain abscesses, but the treatment may not be fully effective because of the difficulty in getting enough of the drug to the site of the infection. Often surgery is required to eliminate the abscess. In these operations, the surgeon lays open the abscess, removes the accumulated fluid and damaged tissue and treats the infection. The chances of recovery usually are good.

Meningitis

The meninges are the membranes that enclose the brain and the upper spinal cord. Meningitis, or infection of the meninges, can be caused by any number of germs, but the most common cause is the meningococcus; sometimes, the infection is a complication of a disease such as influenza or pneumonia.

In meningitis, the membranes become inflamed, producing a number of alarming symptoms: fever, nausea, vomiting, delirium, even coma. Extreme stiffness of the neck, muscle rigidity and arched back may also occur. The headache of meningitis is severe and extremely painful. It is aggravated by physical effort, such as bending and stooping. Often, it is one of the leading symptoms of the infection.

Meningitis once was equivalent to a death sentence for most patients. Antibiotics have changed the picture dramatically, bringing the death rate down to 5 per cent or lower. Recently Army researchers have taken another major step against the disease, which often is endemic in recruit training camps because of the crowding together of large numbers of young men who are suddenly exposed to the germs that cause meningitis. In an effort to prevent epidemics which have hit many Army camps, scientists have developed a vaccine that is effective against one of the most common strains of meningococcus. After large-scale testing, the vaccine was put into use in 1970 in a number of army camps.

Aneurysm

An aneurysm can be compared to a weak spot in an inner tube. As the tube is blown up, the weak spot begins to bulge because it is unable to take the pressure. Too much inflation and the weak spot gives way, puncturing the tube.

In exactly the same way, an aneurysm is a weak spot in the wall of a blood vessel. Unable to take the constant push caused by the heart's contraction, the aneurysm bulges out until it can resemble a bubble in the artery wall. If such an aneurysm occurs in one of the blood vessels of the brain—which is fortunately a rare occurrence—its pressure can cause a headache.

Often, that headache may seem to be the result of migraine. It comes on suddenly, affects only one side of the head, throbs insistently and rises to a peak quickly. One telltale symptom of an aneurysm is the failure of ergotamine to relieve the headache, as would happen if migraine were really the problem. Other signs of aneurysm are the symptoms caused by pressure on the brain: visual defects, partial paralysis and the like. But definite diagnosis of the aneurysm often requires a series of tests, including a skull X-ray. In this procedure, a dye is injected into the blood vessels of the head, so that the X-ray will show any unusual accumulation of dye caused by blood pooling in the aneurysm.

Closely related to the headaches caused by aneurysms, and resembling them, are the headaches due to angiomas—abnormal enlargements of blood vessels that are caused by malformations. The same throbbing pain and difficulties caused by interference with brain function occur in angiomas and aneurysms.

In some cases, the fault in the blood vessels may be repairable by surgery. Most of the time, however, there is little that the physician can do, since the aneurysm may be in an unreachable area. It is not uncommon for an aneurysm or angioma to be discovered only after the blood vessel gives way, causing a hemorrhage.

Hemorrhage

When a blood vessel in the head breaks, whether because of aneurysm, angioma, or simply because an old, stiff artery wall gives way, blood spills out into the brain tissue. Since there is no place for it to go, the blood begins pressing on the brain. What happens then depends on two things: the size of the hemorrhage and its location.

If it is a large hemorrhage, the outlook is exceedingly grave. Death is only a matter of hours or days away. It may be remembered that Franklin D. Roosevelt died from a cerebral hemorrhage, and that his last words were, "I have a terrific headache." Roosevelt slumped into unconsciousness within moments. He died a few hours later.

If the hemorrhage is smaller, the result is a stroke— a loss of bodily function caused by the death of one part of the brain. The extent of the loss depends on the extent of damage. A stroke can cause complete paralysis or it can be so small as to cause only minor problems with speech and vision. The outlook is not always hopeless in these cases. Winston Churchill, Roosevelt's wartime companion in arms, suffered several strokes in the postwar period. Each time, he regained almost complete control again, so that he was able to go on governing England at an age when most of his countrymen were long in retirement.

The headache caused by a hemorrhage is violent, steady and sudden, affecting the entire head. It is often accompanied by paralysis, and disturbances of consciousness. The patient may slump to the floor or go immediately into a coma. When such a hemorrhage occurs, there is little that a physician can do but provide supportive measures for the patient; the outcome is up to the patient's recuperative powers. If the hemorrhage is small, the physician may prescribe drugs designed to prevent further hemorrhages.

Head Injuries

Everyone knows that a hard knock on the head usually causes a headache. So it is probably surprising to learn that these headaches are not purely physical in cause. Even though the cause and effect relationship appears clear, many physicians believe that the blow to the head is often just an excuse that allows deep-seated emotional difficulties to surface in the form of a headache.

Of course, there can be a purely physical headache caused by a blow to the head. In a few cases, the blow may cause an infection that leads to an abscess. In other cases, blood vessels in the head may be damaged so much that they start to hemorrhage slowly. This is very dangerous, since hemorrhage can cause paralysis or death. In still other cases, an injury to the upper part of the spine can result in stiffness that leads to a typical muscle contraction headache.

The headaches caused by these injuries are identical to those resulting from similar, non-injury causes; any abscess produces its typical steady pain, any hemorrhage causes its sudden headache (which should be reported immediately to a physician), and so on. But the headache produced by the combination of a head injury and emotional problems is a different breed of cat. It goes on and on, often characterized by a vague but persistent feeling of pressure in the head. The patient may feel unexplainably weak or dizzy, with frequent complaints about personality problems. The complaints may go on for months or years, making everyone in the family miserable.

Of course, a judicious course of informal psychotherapy by the family physician is a prime requisite for clearing up this kind of headache. But there is another,

91

more unusual, prescription: settle the lawsuit. Physicians have found that accidents, such as automobile accidents, often lead to suits for damages, and that the law case may absorb the interest of the patient to such an extent that the headaches take firmer hold. Only when the lawsuit ends will the patient acknowledge that his headaches have disappeared. Meanwhile, the folks at home have the job of coping with the headaches and assorted symptoms that somehow satisfy the patient's inner needs. The physician in these cases tries to help by prescribing mild pain-killers and by gently steering the patient away from the topic of the accident and the lawsuit.

This does not mean that people who have been in an accident should stoically avoid a physician and assume that a headache will vanish in short order. A doctor should examine anyone who has suffered a head injury, just to make sure that no serious damage has been done. A day or so in bed often is advisable to help clear up a minor headache. It's when the headache hangs on long after the physician can find any physical explanation for it that he will start to look for an underlying emotional reason.

Epilepsy

As has already been mentioned, there is an undefined relationship between migraine and epilepsy. What both conditions have in common is a disturbance of brain function to some extent—much more serious in epilepsy than in migraine. It does appear that epilepsy patients are more prone to have headaches than are persons without the disease, and that migraine and epilepsy are found in the same people more often than would be expected by pure chance. While the full significance of the often confusing and sometimes contradictory findings about these two conditions is not known, some researchers believe that the relationship will lead to fuller knowledge about both epilepsy and migraine.

12.
Neuralgia

NEURALGIA—PAIN ARISING from the nerves—can occur anywhere in the body. When it occurs in the nerves of the head, it produces a headache, one of the most excruciating known. The most prevalent of these cranial neuralgias, trigeminal neuralgia, entered the medical literature during the Middle Ages under the vividly descriptive name of *tortura facies*—facial torture. Through the centuries, until little more than a decade ago, that torture remained almost untouched by the advance of medical knowledge.

Today, however, trigeminal neuralgia can be described as one of the triumphs of modern medical research. Within the past decade, drugs have become available that give relief from the torture to three of every four patients. There are other cranial neuralgias waiting to be conquered, but one research triumph raises hope of more to come.

Trigeminal Neuralgia

There are twelve pairs of cranial nerves. These lead

from the brain to other parts of the head and upper body. They include the optic nerve (vision), the olefactory nerve (smell), and so forth. Over the centuries, these nerves have been numbered and their functions outlined in endless detail, but they still have a few mysteries.

The fifth pair of cranial nerves are the trigeminals. They exit from the head through small holes in the back of the skull, branching off in three trunks to the front of the head. Among other functions, they control the chewing muscles, contribute to the sense of taste, and supply the sensory function for much of the face.

For a reason that is still not fully understood, the trigeminal nerve sometimes goes haywire. Without warning, a person is hit by brief piercing jabs of violent, almost unendurable pain. The pain comes in spurts, each lasting from a few seconds to a few minutes, vanishing as suddenly as it comes. These attacks may occur in clusters, which can occur as often as twenty or thirty times a day. (Because of this, and because the pain usually is confined to one side of the face, trigeminal neuralgia sometimes is mistaken for cluster headache.) The names given to trigeminal neuralgia testify to the intensity of the pain; many physicians still call it *tic doloreux,* literally "painful tic." Patients describe the pain as burning, shooting or dartlike, as if a knife were being thrust into the face. Any portion of the face supplied by the trigeminal nerves can be affected—the cheek, the lower jaw, the eye, or the forehead; in some patients, the pain strikes in different places during different clusters.

The attacks can be caused by a number of apparently innocuous factors. Just touching a certain point on the face may do it, or the normal motions of chewing, talking, washing the face or brushing the teeth, or eating ice cream, or being out in the cold, to mention a few of many causes. Naturally, the trigeminal neuralgia patient will tend to lead a rather careful and guarded life for fear of setting off one of the familiar, excruciating attacks.

A few years ago, any description of trigeminal neuralgia would have ended on a fairly gloomy note, with the description of a few not-too-effective measures that constituted the entire medical arsenal against this unhappy condition. Today, it's different. Thanks to the intuition of a medical researcher and some effective scientific spadework, effective drugs are available for most patients.

The key observation was that a compound called carbamazepine suppressed the nerve reflexes in the part of the face served by the trigeminal nerves. Someone then got the inspired idea that the drug would be effective against trigeminal neuralgia—and he was right. Long years of animal testing and then clinical trials on people followed, and carbamezepine now is available under the trade name Tegretol, marketed in the United States by Geigy Pharmaceuticals.

Carbamazepine is not a drug to fool around with. It has been known to cause serious, potentially fatal, cases of anemia and other blood disorders. Physicians are advised to keep monitoring their patient's blood when the drug is prescribed. Offsetting these side effects is the relief given by carbamazepine—relief in twenty-four to forty-eight hours for as many as three of every four trigeminal neuralgia patients. In a situation where previous treatments were both slower and much less effective, these results are revolutionary. Carbamazepine is taken daily to prevent attacks. Physicians will try to give the lowest dose possible and to reduce or eliminate the drug periodically in order to minimize the occurrence of adverse side effects.

If carbamazepine doesn't start working within four days, the physician will start adding other drugs to the prescription. Usually, those drugs will be anticonvulsants that are prescribed for epilepsy. In fact, some physicians prefer to use anticonvulsants —notably Dilantin, perhaps the most popular drug for epilepsy—before they try carbamazepine, because of carbamazepine's severe side effects. What the anticonvulsants and carbamazepine have in common is the ability to interrupt some re-flex activities of the spinal cord and brain stem (the lowest part of the brain). By studying the action of these drugs on the brain, researchers have been able to get a better picture of the cause of trigeminal neuralgia. This is an excellent example of how one inspired medical advance opens the way for even greater advances. The better scientists understand a disease, the more weapons they will be able to develop against it.

Because there are a number of drugs available, the physician often will experiment until he finds just the right combination for a specific patient. Sometimes, however, there is no right combination. When a patient cannot get relief from drugs, or when serious side effects make it necessary to discontinue drug treatment, the physician will fall back on the treatments developed in pre-drug time.

One such treatment is injection of alcohol into the trigeminal nerve at the point where it leaves the skull. This can provide relief for months or even years, but the effects of the injection wear off in the end. Another injection gives renewed relief, but for a shorter time. The cycle of injections can go on, each shot giving briefer relief, until finally the alcohol fails to work at all. The patient then is back where he started, except that he has had a fairly prolonged period free from attacks of trigeminal neuralgia.

The preferred treatment in case the drugs fail is surgery, in which the problem is ended by cutting the trigeminal nerve. This is a safe, usually uncomplicated procedure. Its main drawback is the loss of function in the nerve, which means that the sense of touch in the affected area is lost. Most patients find this numbness easier to live with than the periodic attacks of trigeminal neuralgia. In recent years, steps have been taken to eliminate even this drawback. Working with extreme care and modern electronic equipment, surgeon Yoshio Hosibuchi of the University of California Medical Center in San Francisco has developed a method of carefully singling out the specific parts of the nerve that are affected by neuralgia. Those parts are inactivated, while the rest of the nerve is left intact. Dr. Hosobuchi reports that this technique eliminates the pain while retaining much of the nerve's functions, so that patients can be pain-free without a numb face.

All in all, the trigeminal neuralgia story is one of the happier pages in recent medical history. The advances made in both drug therapy and surgical treatment are textbook examples of the everyday benefits that are derived from the dollars spent on medical research.

Glossopharyngeal Neuralgia

As trigeminal neuralgia affects the fifth cranial nerve, glossopharyngeal neuralgia affects the ninth cranial nerve, which goes to the back of the mouth, part of the ear, and the interior of the neck. Glossopharyngeal neuralgia is much rarer than trigeminal neuralgia; for every 100 cases of trigeminal neuralgia, there is one case of glossopharyngeal neuralgia. The pain has the same severe, stabbing qualities, but it is confined to the throat and mouth in most cases, which makes it easier to distinguish.

The same drugs and techniques use for trigeminal neuralgia are equally effective for ninth nerve neuralgia—carbamazepine, the anticonvulsants used for epilepsy, and so on. If these fail, surgery is the usual treatment. Cutting the nerve ends the pain effectively.

Atypical Neuralgias

Why do doctors use such awkward language to describe ailments? Patients whose tongues stumble over such phrases as "trigeminal neuralgia" and "atypical neuralgia" often ask that question. The reason (aside from a certain professional snobbery that afflicts almost every trade, not only medicine) is that these seemingly awkward phrases are actually quite precise and descriptive. "Trigeminal neuralgia" is pain of the fifth nerve, and

"atypical neuralgia" are just what the name de-
scribes—neuralgias that are not of the typical kind. The
phrase is kind of a grab-bag for various conditions, but it
does enable doctors to put a number of similar conditions under a single descriptive heading.

Lumping them together has one major advantage: it
corresponds to the reality that a physician runs into
when he tries to make a precise diagnosis of one of these
neuralgias. "Clear-cut differentiation of these conditions may be difficult, if not impossible, and there is
considerable argument among specialists in the neurological disciplines as to the firm establishment of any
of these syndromes as definite clinical entities," says Dr.
Patrick D. Kenan of the Duke University Medical Center.

There are a number of features distinguishing the atypical neuralgias from the neuralgias of the fifth or ninth
nerve. The major distinction is the nature of the pain.
Instead of being episodic, brief and darting, it is steady
and aching, often spreading over much of the head, perhaps lasting for several days. There are no "trigger
points," or sore spots that can set off attacks. Instead of
being confined to the area served by one cranial nerve, the
pain can occur in areas served by several. And severing
either the fifth or the ninth cranial nerves does nothing to
relieve the pain.

One such atypical neuralgia goes by the imposing name
of sphenopalatine ganglion neuralgia—again, a seemingly confusing name that is actually precise and
descriptive; it refers to neuralgia of a specific nerve structure found in the rear of the nasal cavity. This condition
produces a burning pain over one side of the cheek, which
can spread to the neck and shoulder. Alcohol injections
can do some good for the condition, but they cannot end
it permanently.

There is a relatively long list of atypical neuralgias,
most of them fairly rare. They can lead physicians a mer-
ry chase before they are diagnosed, because of their resem-

blance to migraine or other cranial neuralgias. Once diagnosed, they are not easy to treat. Physicians are still waiting for a research breakthrough in this area.

Neuritis

Aside from the essentially unexplained neuralgias, the nerves are also subject to the same kind of problems that other parts of the body suffer from—infection, growths, and so on. For example, herpes virus infection of a cranial nerve can produce a steady, burning pain that persists for months, until the infection goes away. Treatment is limited to prescribing pain-killers and assuring the patient that the neuritis is bound to end sooner or later.

Tumors are most likely to affect the fifth, ninth and tenth cranial nerves, causing a deep ache. Sometimes neuritis is caused by a growth of the nerve itself, called a neuroma. Removal of the tumor by surgery is the preferred method of treatment.

13.

A Miscellany of Headaches

THIS CHAPTER MAY help patients appreciate just what the physician has to face when someone walks into his office complaining about a pain in the head. It's already been made clear that diagnosis of even the common forms of headache can be a difficult job. This chapter will add a number of other pains in the head that complicate the job.

The Ear

Physicians draw a careful distinction between ear pain and earache. Ear pain can be caused by ailments that have nothing to do with the ear. Because a number of cranial nerves pass through the region of the ear, a condition that affects a different part of these nerves may manifest itself as a pain in the ear. That's why the physician may look down your mouth when you come in complaining of a painful ear.

Earache is a different story. Generally, it is caused by

infection of the ear. Summertime is the peak season for ear infections, since people are out in the open during warm days, swimming to get exercise and lying on the grass. Warmth and moisture breed infectious agents, such as bacteria and fungi.

The earache of such an infection does the patient a favor if it brings him to the physician's office. Doctors always pay careful attention to any infection near the brain, because the infection can turn from a mild bother to a possibly fatal illness by spreading just a short distance. Prompt treatment by antibiotics and other drugs is the usual course of action. Before such drugs existed, surgery was often necessary to avoid loss of hearing or brain abscesses arising from ear infections. Today, there is no longer a crisis atmosphere surrounding an ear infection—once treatment is begun. That's why it is important not to neglect any pain in the ear, especially a mild pain that seems to increase from day to day. It may be a sign of a growing infection, or of an inflammation caused by a cold. Neglected, either one can cause a lot more trouble than most people realize. See the doctor.

The Teeth

Most Americans tend to think of their teeth as pain-producing mechanisms—and the only time they *do* think of their teeth is when a toothache is in full swing. If any kind of emotional problem is added to this tendency, and a headache is thrown in, the results may be disastrous to a perfectly healthy mouthful of teeth.

It was not uncommon in the past for patients to have all their teeth pulled as a measure to relieve chronic headaches. This did occasionally work, but almost invariably because of the psychological effect of the procedure, not because of anything that was wrong with the teeth.

There are occasions when a headache is caused by tooth trouble—for example, where tooth decay is severe enough to start affecting the sinus in which the root of the tooth is imbedded, or when the nerves that throb because of the toothache transmit the pain to other parts of the head. But the proper treatment of this headache is not to pull all the teeth; it is elimination of the tooth decay in the specific teeth involved, followed by regular visits to the dentist and tooth care to insure that decay does not recur.

Malocclusion—severe misalignment of the teeth—may sometimes be bad enough to cause headaches. Dentists have a variety of techniques, including surgery for the worst cases, to correct malocclusion. Unhappily, malocclusion sometimes causes emotional problems because of its effect on the appearance of the patient, and those problems may lead to tension headaches. At this point, what started as a dental problem has turned into something else. In addition to correcting the actual malocclusion, the dentist must do something about the patient's self-image. But to blame these headaches on dental problems is really stretching the meaning of the word "dental."

In short, the teeth are vastly overrated as causes of headaches. The pain usually is in the mind, not the teeth, of the patient.

Constipation Headache

This is another headache that really isn't—an entirely imaginary head pain caused by a beautiful theory that is totally untrue.

The theory runs like this: The role of the large intestine is to collect and dispose of the solid waste products of the body. It stands to reason that these waste products contain harmful substances. Therefore, the longer the period that the waste products remain in the intestine, the more of these poisons filter back into the body, causing a variety of troubles, including headache. Finally, it also stands to reason that the only way to prevent this "autointoxication" is to move the bowels regularly. A day without a bowel movement, according to this theory, is a day in which the body is poisoned steadily.

There's only one thing wrong with this theory: everything. Careful study has established beyond doubt that nothing poisonous is absorbed into the body from the large intestines, no matter how long the time period between bowel movements. Equally careful studies have also established the fact that one bowel movement a day is by no means the rule for every person. Some people are perfectly healthy and happy with a bowel movement every other day, or even every third day.

The problem is that people who take constipation seriously are in no mood to listen to scientific facts. These people know that they are constipated—don't ask them why, they just know. They also know that they have frequent headaches. Ergo, the headaches are caused by the constipation. Since magazine and television advertisements are subtly tailored to encourage such beliefs, many of these people become first-class consumers of laxatives, jumping from one to another in hopes of finding the product that will give them perfect regularity.

Alas, there is no such thing to be found on any store shelf. The emotions govern the intestines as much as they govern all other organs of the body, and nervousness, anxiety, a sudden change in diet, or any one of a thousand other factors can cause a change in bowel habits. Since many of these factors also cause headache, people suffering from both find the cause and effect relationship too logical to resist, especially because it is so comforting psychologically.

Some people do have the need for laxatives, but it is always a temporary need, and the laxatives should be taken on the advice of a physician. For the real relief of the problem, the physician will recommend a regular diet and a calm mind. For those people who are unable to accept this line of reasoning, the informal psychotherapy that is so often the stock in trade of the family physician can do more than a railroad car full of laxatives.

Hypoglycemia Headaches

Everyone has heard of diabetes, the disease that is characterized by an oversupply of sugar in the blood. Fewer have heard of hypoglycemia, the condition in which there is a shortage of blood sugar. Since sugar provides energy for the body, a shortage can cause various difficulties, including a headache.

In most normal people, hypoglycemia will occur only when something prevents an adequate intake of food. That "something" could be simply a skipped meal or two. Or it could be brought on by one of the crash diets that weight-conscious Americans are apt to try in an effort to take off a few pounds quickly. Some people suffer from an overproduction of insulin, which means that sugar will be consumed at a faster rate. Even diabetics can suffer from low blood sugar if they take too much insulin or other antidiabetic medicine.

For persons with no diabetes or other abnormality, hypoglycemia generally occurs just before mealtime. It produces weakness and trembling, with a dull headache that seems to suffuse the entire head, and a quite natural feeling of hunger. Eating usually eliminates the headaches and the other symptoms. If a good meal doesn't work, then it's time for a visit to the doctor to see whether hyperinsulinism—overproduction of insulin—is to blame.

For most people, irregular eating habits are enough explanation for the hypoglycemic headache. The tendency for many people to skip a meal—breakfast for most young people, lunch for the busy executive—and to diet rigidly and irregularly can throw the body off enough to start a headache. Regular meals will eliminate the hypoglycemic headache in all but a few instances. If they don't work, it is not advisable to try to build up the body's sugar supply by eating sweets. Aside from the possibility that the self-diagnosis might be wrong, hyperinsulinism calls for a medically determined diet and careful supervision by the family physician. There is one incidental benefit that many people will reap from correcting hypoglycemia: since the condition tends to make people unusually irritable, eliminating it may help end family squabbles that can often lead to tension headaches—two kinds of relief for the price of one.

Hangover Headache

Once upon a time, a medical researcher who was studying the hangover set about it in an entirely scientific manner. Gathering a group of volunteers together, he gave them carefully controlled doeses of alcohol until they were clearly tipsy. Waiting a few hours, he then began studying them for signs of hangover.

But there were no such signs. Without exception, the scientific drinkers were clear-eyed, jolly, steady-handed and headache-free. Despite their heavy consumption of alcohol, none of them had hangovers.

Instead of writing off the experiment as a total loss, the scientist described it as a success, because he had made a basic discovery: It's not really alcohol that causes the hangover. It's alcohol plus the social ingredients that go into drinking. Since that pivotal experiment, other researchers have filled in the details.

To start with, whiskey doesn't contain just alcohol. It also has ingredients called congeners, which gave it taste, color, flavor and aroma. (Vodka contains almost no congeners, which accounts for its lack of color and taste as well as its reputation of being hangover-free.) While scientists have a good picture of what alcohol does to the system, they know almost nothing about the effects of the congeners—except that they very likely contribute to the hangover.

Then again, most people drink alcohol at parties where chatter and music tend to be loud at the start and louder as partygoers become more lubricated. The snacks handed around at parties are tempting and filling, but hardly well-balanced nutritionally. As for alcohol itself, it has several effects. Alcohol increases the blood rate and heart pressure. It dilates blood vessels, which accounts for the rosy glow drinkers seem to have; the small blood vessels in the skin are dilated, increasing the supply of blood near the surface and giving people a ruddy look. Alcohol is a diuretic, increasing the amount of fluid excreted by the body to such an extent that the drinker becomes somewhat dehydrated.

And finally, alcohol relaxes the brain's filter system, which ordinarily screens out excess stimuli, so that a torrent of sounds and sights come flooding in unchecked.

That's great the night before—but oh, the morning after! When hangover arrives, its headache is perhaps the worst part of it. Hangover produces a throbbing headache, beating in time with the pulse. It is a vascular headache caused by overdilated blood vessels, and it is made worse by changes in position and even minor jolts, such as those caused by coughs and sneezes. Walking is an effort, running is out of the question, and noise is unbearable. To top it off are the other symptoms: furry tongue caused by dehydration, queasiness caused by disturbance of the brain center that controls vomiting, indigestion caused by unwise eating.

Knowing the cause of the hangover helps physicians prescribe a cure. Some things can be done the night before, such as sticking to vodka during the party and an avoidance of overeating. To help the body metabolize the alcohol better, it helps to supply it with fructose, a form of sugar that induces the body to burn alcohol faster. Fresh fruits are rich in fructose, as is honey. A slice of toast with honey just before retiring, or a glass of fruit juice on awakening can help speed recovery. A cup of black coffee is also a help, since it contains caffeine that will constrict the dilated arteries. For really serious hangovers, ergotamine can be tried, but only on a physician's recommendation.

For dehydration, water alone won't do, since it will not correct the mineral imbalance caused by fluid loss. Something salty, such as beef broth, will supply a fluid that more closely fits the body's needs. Broth will also supply calories for fitness. Finally, lying down with an ice bag on the head is wrong—the ice bag constricts the dilated arteries, but lying down tends to keep them dilated. An erect posture, difficult as it may be to achieve, will do more good. And, of course, don't try alcohol as a hangover cure. The hair of the dog is likely to bite hard, compounding the problems.

That's the light side of hangover headache. The serious

side is the recurring hangover, which means that someone is drinking too much too frequently. Alcoholism is a disease whose proportions are just beginning to be realized. At least four million Americans suffer from alcoholism, and the losses in money and lives and the grief are almost incalculable. Simple preventive measures and morning-after treatment are fine for the person who gets an occasional hangover—and who doesn't? For the person who gets frequent hangovers, attention to the emotional and physical factors behind them is essential.

Toxic Headaches

After centuries of neglecting what industrialism was doing to the environment and to people, we have awakened to the harm done by pollution. We now know that we may literally be poisoning the world to such an extent that the human race may not survive. Workers are becoming aware that the toxic materials used in many industrial processes, and in the home as well, can do serious damage. Inhaling or otherwise ingesting these substances can, among other things, cause headaches. The headaches should be welcomed, because they give warning of more serious troubles.

To list all the substances that have been implicated as hazards to health would take a fat volume. There are gases, liquids and dusts galore, and it's almost impossible to escape from all of them.

For instance, a short time ago, workers in the tunnels leading into New York City began to complain loudly about the high levels of carbon monoxide that they were forced to breathe on their posts—levels so elevated that prolonged exposure could produce lasting damage. The average motorist probably shrugged in sympathy and let it go at that. But it is the fumes from the average motorist's automobile that contain the carbon monoxide, and a faulty muffler or exhaust system can expose a driver to all the problems that the tunnel workers complained about—headache, nausea, dizziness and abdominal pain, among others. Many drivers who finish a day on the road with a splitting headache attribute the pain to eyestrain. They might be better off to check the fumes coming from the exhaust pipe. And in some cities, it's not even necessary to be a driver. Just standing on a busy corner and breathing the polluted air may be enough to get a headache going.

Sometimes what looks like an occupational headache that is limited to a small group of workers turns out to have a much wider significance. Such is the case with "munition worker headaches," caused by inhalation of nitrites and so called because these chemicals are used in making ammunition.

But nitrites are also used to treat angina pectoris, a common form of heart disease characterized by sudden attacks of severe pain. These attacks come when arteries clamp down, severely limiting the flow of blood. Nitrites dilate blood vessels, and so are used to bring relief from angina attacks. Physicians have found that relief from angina via nitrite treatment often means increased frequency and severity of migraine headaches, caused by more dilation of the cranial blood vessels. The physician must then decide whether one form of pain can be traded off against the other.

Until recently, carbon tetrachloride was a fairly common ingredient in cleaning fluids for home and industrial use. Inhaling small amounts of carbon tetrachloride can cause a headache. Inhaling large amounts can be fatal. Over the protests of some manufacturers, the federal government acted to ban carbon tetrachloride products from the home.

Another example of unknowing pollution was discovered in 1970, when studies showed unduly high levels of mercury in the waters of most states. Mercury is a poison that, in addition to causing headaches, can cause brain damage or even death. After federal officials moved on the issue, a number of manufacturers quickly cut down the amount of mercury that was pouring out of their factories with the waste water. But that was not in time to prevent a ban on eating fish from a number of rivers and lakes where the mercury content was too high for safety.

In the past, it was possible to say that only workers in industries that handled such substances as mercury and arsonic in large quantities had to worry about the headaches these substances cause. Now, however, it begins to appear that no one is totally safe. Globally, this problem of pollution could be mankind's number one headache.

Spinal Puncture Headache

In some cases, physicians find it necessary to remove a small amount of fluid from the spinal column to help make a diagnosis. The fluid that is being examined surrounds both the spinal column and the brain, floating them gently to help cushion against shocks.

When the needle is inserted, often more spinal fluid leaks out than is intended. If enough fluid is lost, the brain drops lower within the skull. As it does so, it pulls gently but insistently—and painfully—on the arteries and other structures attached to it. That causes a spinal puncture headache. Since it takes days for the body to manufacture enough new fluid to bring the body back to its normal level, the headache may last for days. If the patient can lie flat, there will be little or no pain. But since most people do spend most of their time upright, the spinal puncture headache can be a decided nuisance while it lasts. Fortunately, relatively few people require spinal taps, so the spinal puncture headache is a decided rarity.

Women and Men

For some women, menstruation automatically means headache—a fact that has produced a large and thriving industry whose product is patent medicines for the female trade. Nothing that anyone says will stop production of these medications, but physicians say that aspirin, rest and a hot-water bottle or ice pack can do just as good a job. As for the crankiness and emotional upsets that so often accompany menstruation, and which may contribute to the

109

headache, a little understanding on the part of husband and wife goes a long way.

That may not be enough for the menopause, the time of life when the production of female sex hormones is reduced dramatically. This is a time of serious stress, both mental and physical, and often medical attention is required. Many physicians now accept the theory that some of the symptoms of menopause are unnecessary and avoidable. These physicians will prescribe regular doses of female sex hormones to reduce the physical changes and mental bothers of menopause. Often, they will prescribe tranquillizers or antidepressants to tide the patient over.

What most people don't realize is that there is a male menopause, also. Usually, the male menopause does not occur as suddenly and drastically as the female menopause. Instead, there is a long period during which the hormonal output of the male changes, slowly but steadily. As this happens, the attitudes and behavior of the man can change drastically—no surprise, considering the well-known link between the hormones and the emotions. The emotional stress created by the male menopause may lead to a series of tension headaches or other manifestations. Some observers believe that the tendency of men in their fifties to start running around with much younger women is a result of the physical and emotional changes caused by the male menopause. According to this theory, the man feels his masculinity ebbing away and makes a grab for one last fling. Whatever the truth is, simply knowing that there is such a thing as the male menopause and understanding its effects can help the situation considerably.

The Sun

The sun is fun, but overdoing it can cause heat exhaustion or sunstroke. It's not the light of the sun but the heat that's responsible. The body gets so hot that its heat-regulating system goes out of order. Weakness, dizziness, profuse sweating and unconsciousness can result. In severe cases, the person can die before help becomes available.

The headache of overexposure to the sun is caused in part by the loss of body fluids through perspiration. Getting the patient out of the sun, loosening his clothing, and giving an ice pack when possible will meet the immediate emergency. The headache will then ebb of its own accord. Prevention is simple: avoid overexposure, either by getting out of the sun entirely or by wearing a hat.

14.

Summing Up

THE TWO THEMES that recur again and again in this volume are the diversity of causes for headache and the advisability of consulting a doctor for most recurrent or severe headaches. Those two themes are intertwined, because if headaches all had the same cause and the same treatment, there would be little need to see a physician. As it is, it takes the skill of the physician to select from the multiplicity of possible causes the one real cause of his patient's headache, and the one specific treatment that will bring relief from the headaches.

This being so, the patient who brings his headache problem to the family doctor should be ready with information that the doctor will need. Some of the information will concern the headache itself. It may take a long series of detailed questions to gather all the information required to make the diagnosis. How often do the headaches occur? Is the pain throbbing or steady? What part of the head does the pain strike? Do the headaches occur any particular time of day? How long do they last? Have they just begun or have they been occurring in the past? Are there any incidents in particular that always bring on a headache? The questions will go on and on, as the doctor forms a tentative diagnosis and then gathers the information he will need to prove or disprove his theory.

A patient should also be prepared to answer what seem like personal questions. Is everything all right on the job? Is family life serene or tumultuous? Are the children causing a lot of trouble? Is there a family history of headache? Did you have headaches when you were a child? All of these are as essential as the other kind of question in most cases when the physician faces the challenge of a headache.

That's because of a paradox. Underlying the obvious diversity of headaches is a common thread—the emotions. Sooner or later, the physician expects to find an emotional basis for the great majority of headaches that he must treat. Even when the headache has a purely physical cause, the emotional attitude of the patient can determine the severity and length of the suffering. A happy man or a contented woman will take in stride pain that will cause endless bother to a person whose personal problems seem insoluble.

This means that the physician must be a little more than a physician: he must be a psychotherapist and a counselor as well. Much of the relief he provides will come not from medicines but from helping the patient understand the real causes of the headaches. Even when he prescribes pain-killers, his real goal may be accomplished more in the way that he treats the patient than by the action of the drugs.

This is a concept that many people refused to believe. In part, we still are in the throes of the reaction against the belief that medieval ideas, such as the laying on of hands, were more than just superstitions. Until fairly recently, physicians looked only for physical causes of diseases. Now that research has made clear the relationship between the mind and the body, it is once more acceptable to believe that purely psychological factors can produce diseases.

But physicians do not rely on that concept alone. New

drugs and surgical techniques are being created constantly for treatment of headaches. Long years of research have laid a firm foundation on which major new advances can be made. The last ten years have seen the introduction of effective drugs for prevention of migraine, treatment of trigeminal neuralgia and aid to other headaches. Drugs now in the laboratory will extend those advances, and theories that are being tested will point the way toward more effective drug therapies.

Since headache has been with man since the earliest days of civilization, there seems to be little chance that it will vanish now, especially in light of the increased tension that modern society seems to generate. Physicians may not be able, single-handedly, to give their patients the serenity of mind that can prevent many headaches. But physicians can —and do—use the increasingly effective drugs that research has made available for treatment of headaches. It is the combination of medical research and competent physicians that guarantees us the most effective help for our headaches.

Headache Clinics

There are three clinics in the United States devoted exclusively to headache. They are the Headache Clinic of the Mount Sinai Hospital and Medical Center in Chicago; the Headache Unit of the Division of Neurology, Montefiore Hospital and Medical Center in New York; and the Headache Clinic of the University of New Mexico School of Medicine in Albuquerque.

Persons who want information on help available in their area may contact the American Association for the Study of Headache at 5252 Northwestern Avenue, Chicago, Illinois 60625. There is also a National Headache Foundation, with headquarters in Chicago, which is chartered as a nonprofit association for such purposes as issuing a monthly bulletin for headache patients and supporting headache research. This is somewhat modeled after the British Migraine Association, an organization whose financial and moral support has been of major assistance to headache researchers in England.